What They Don't Tell You About

Tell You About

Having a Baby

An Obstetrician's Unofficial Guide to Preconception, Pregnancy, and Postpartum Life

Heather L. Johnson

WHAT THEY DON'T TELL YOU ABOUT HAVING A BABY: AN OBSTETRICIAN'S
UNOFFICIAL GUIDE TO PRECONCEPTION, PREGNANCY, AND POSTPARTUM LIFE

Copyright © 2019 Atlantic Publishing Group, Inc.

1405 SW 6th Avenue • Ocala, Florida 34471 • Phone 352-622-1825 • Fax 352-622-1875
Website: www.atlantic-pub.com • Email: sales@atlantic-pub.com
SAN Number: 268-1250

Library of Congress Cataloging-in-Publication Data

Names: Johnson, Heather, author.
Title: What they don't tell you about having a baby : an obstetrician's unofficial guide to preconception,
    pregnancy, and postpartum life / Heather Johnson.
Description: Ocala, Florida : Atlantic Publishing Group, Inc., [2019] | Includes bibliographical references
    and index.
Identifiers: LCCN 2019024596 (print) | LCCN 2019024597 (ebook) | ISBN 9781620236567 (paper-
    back) | ISBN 9781620236574 (ebook)
Subjects: LCSH: Pregnancy—Popular works. | Childbirth—Popular works. | Prenatal care—Popular
    works.
Classification: LCC RG525 .J63 2019 (print) | LCC RG525 (ebook) | DDC 618.2—dc23
LC record available at https://lccn.loc.gov/2019024596
LC ebook record available at https://lccn.loc.gov/2019024597

Printed in the United States

PROJECT MANAGER: Katie Cline
INTERIOR LAYOUT AND JACKET DESIGN: Nicole Sturk
COVER AND INTERIOR ART: Marcel Trindade

Table of Contents

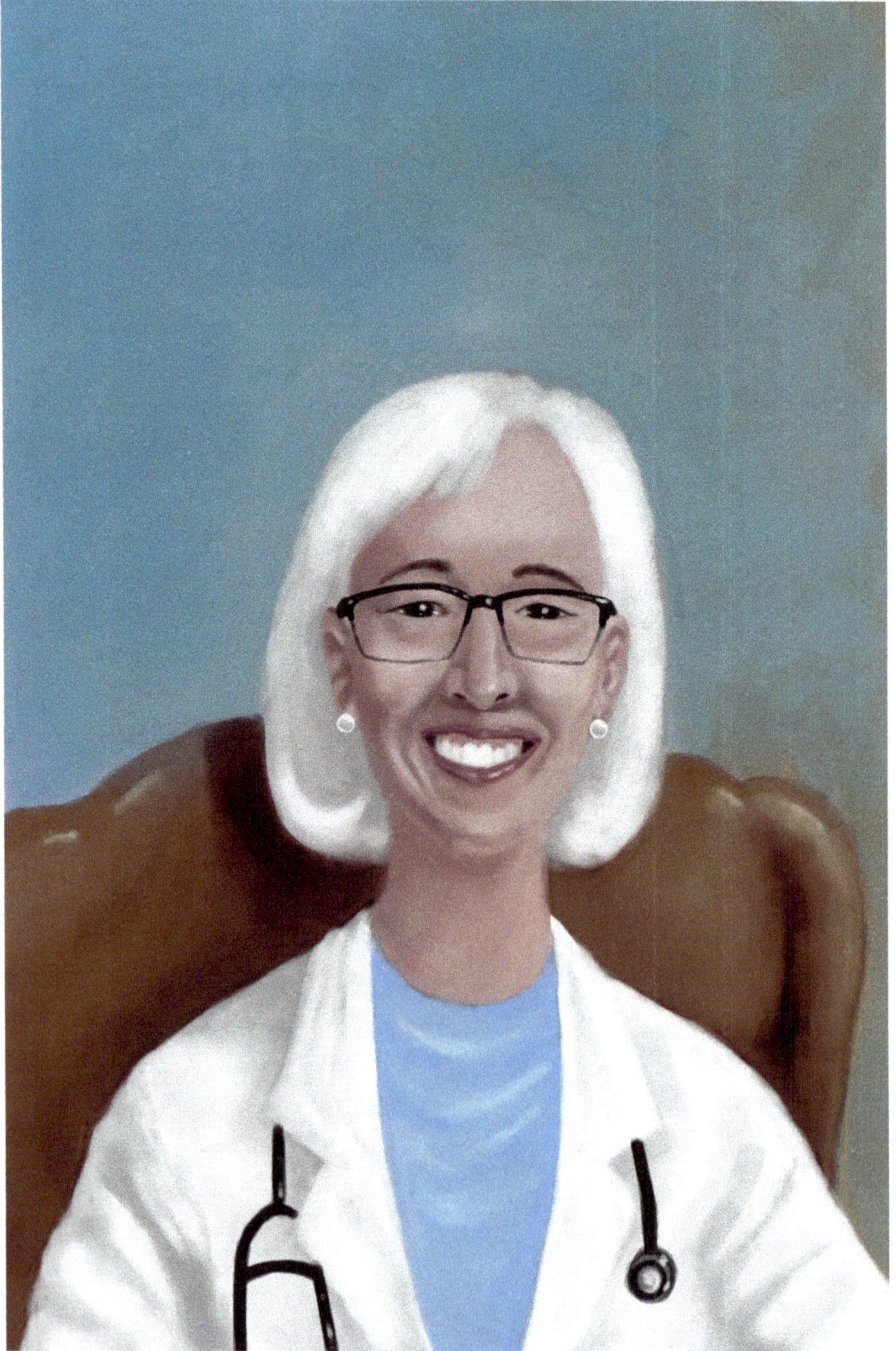

Introduction

On January 12, 2019, I delivered my last baby, Jack David, weighing in at 8 pounds and 10 ounces. After 40 years and over 3,500 babies, I had the privilege of delivering a young lady whom I had known for 32 years, the daughter of one of the most big-hearted, beautiful women I have ever had the pleasure to know.

I was torn then between cracking open a bottle of vintage champagne and toasting my remarkably good fortune or welling up with tears and bemoaning the fact that I would never again be able to participate in this remarkable event. In 40 years, I was never able to get used to this awesome privilege. Until the very last delivery, I continued to be amazed at that tiny, perfect human being who appeared at the end of this miraculous process.

It is not uncommon for me to go to the store or a restaurant in my neighborhood and run into someone whose child I delivered. Not a month goes by when I don't have a patient whose face seems familiar; I look at her last name and then ask, "Was your mother's name such and such?" The smile reveals her mother 30-some-years earlier, and she tells me that I delivered her. What an honor. Such trust. Such respect. I can't begin to say how much this means to me.

Last Mother's Day I received a card from a former patient whose children I had delivered 27 and 25 years ago. She just wanted to let me know that she thought of me often and fondly, and wanted to thank me and provide me with an update on their lives.

I started medical school at Yale University School of Medicine in 1975 fully expecting that I would be a psychiatrist. I was interested in how the mind worked and anxious to help those who needed some direction along their way in life.

Unfortunately, at that time, a sort of snobbery existed in some of the more elite medical schools, and the unstated impression was clearly given that smart people went into internal medicine. The not-so-smart people went into surgery. Pediatrics? "Little people, little minds." I will not try to justify this way of thinking. The world of medicine was different then, and many things have changed for the better. Suffice to say that, at the time, I bought into it. I was smart, wasn't I? Hence my early decision to go into internal medicine. The problem was that I hated it. So many sick people with end-stage diseases that were, in many cases, not necessarily motivated to change their lifestyles. I was young and full of energy and ideals. I wanted results on a faster and more palpable basis.

My obstetrics and gynecology (OB/GYN) clerkship was the last of my third-year rotations. It was a check of the boxes—nothing I was the least bit interested in. To my surprise, I found myself reading the study materials, not because I wanted to look good on rounds, but because I was interested in the subject matter. I enjoyed all the different aspects: the surgery, the office visits with their preventive medicine and personal conversations with the patients, and following women through their labor, delivery, and postpartum periods.

I remember praying that God would let me love radiology or dermatology, fields that would allow me to sleep at night and make a good living at the same time. However, the more time I spent on the wards, the more I loved the OB/GYN rotation.

Fast forward 40 years, and I have had the honor and privilege of delivering literally thousands of babies and coming to know thousands upon thousands of women who have trusted me with their health, both physically and emotionally, often at the most vulnerable time of their lives. I have truly been blessed with my patients and career choice. If you would allow me, I would like to share some of my reflections from a career and a life well lived.

Over the years, the practice of medicine has changed in a number of ways: the demands, the paperwork, the regulations, the malpractice environment, and the cost of education overwhelm many physicians today. I understand and feel their pain. However, none of that overshadows the many rewards I have received from this occupation. I have had the best career.

What follows should not be viewed so much as an official manual for having babies; there are plenty of books that cover this. Rather, it should be looked upon as a compilation of the real conversations I had with my patients and the many lessons I learned along the way, as well as with some of "Dr. J's pearls." The intent is to pass along my observations in the hope that they might be helpful to patients and providers; this book is my version of Dr. Spock's "mind meld" in Star Trek (if you are old enough to know what that means).

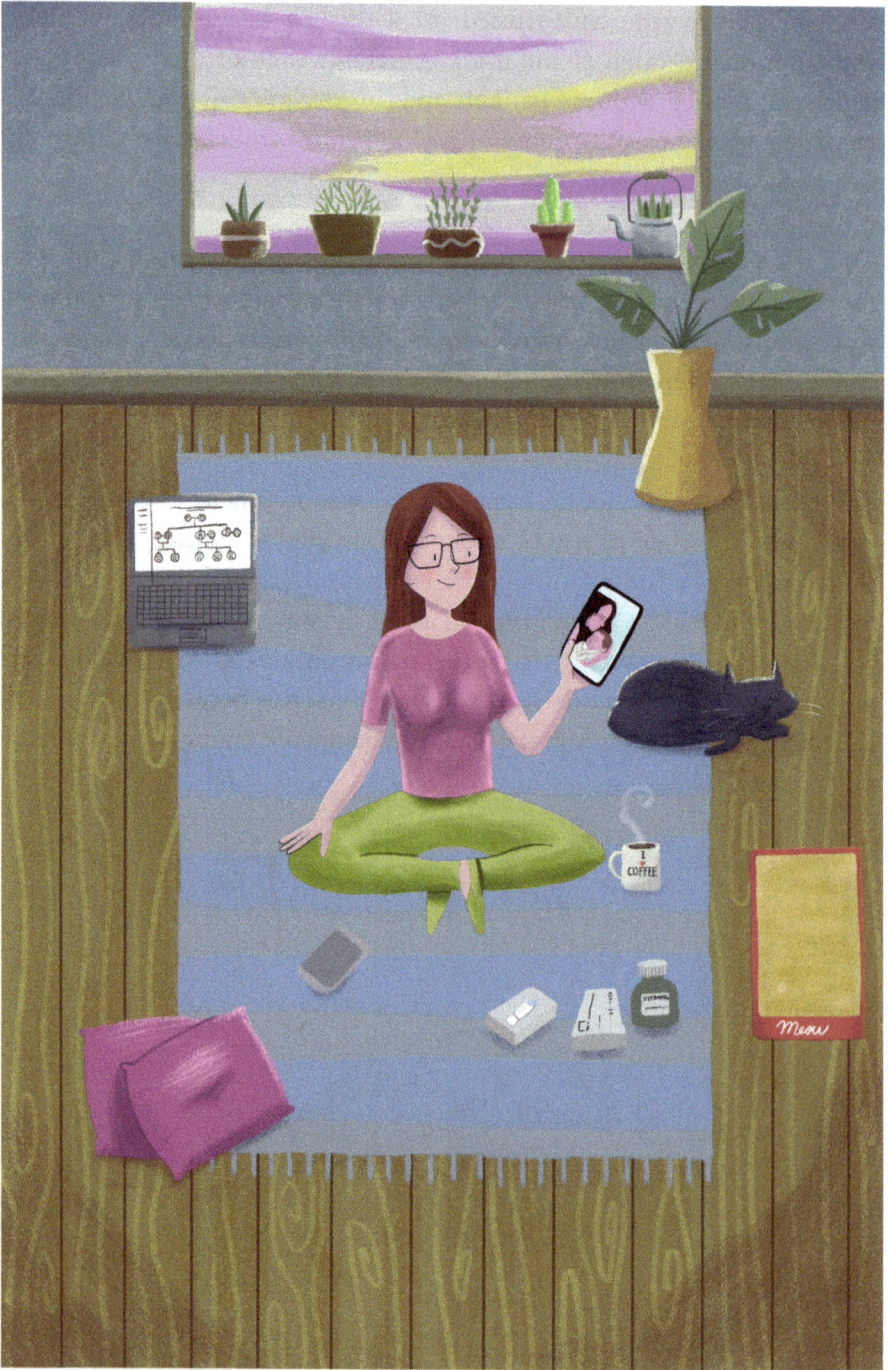

Part One

Preconception Considerations

The Basic Biology of Getting Pregnant

We all remember that we learned about the human reproductive system in high school and college. The problem for many is that they don't remember what they learned. So, just when and how should you try for pregnancy?

The average menstrual cycle is 28 days. In reality, it can range from 25 to 32 days or so without being considered abnormal. Typically, ovulation occurs about 14 days before the onset of the menstrual cycle. In a 28-day cycle, that corresponds to the 14th day from the first day of your last period. If your cycles last for 25 days, you might ovulate as early as day 11. In 32-day cycles, that might not happen until day 21.

If you simply stop using birth control and have intercourse two or three times a week, you have a very good chance of conceiving within a year. If you concentrate intercourse around the probable time of ovulation, you should conceive within a few cycles. Not everyone is equal here though. Teenagers can stand downwind of sperm and get pregnant. A 40-year-old can, and often does, take much longer. This is because the longer a woman lives, the fewer functional eggs she has.

In utero, the female reproductive system is formed in the fifth month, along with the urinary system. The number of eggs in the female fetus is initially over 6 or 7 million. For the remainder of a female's life, there is a monthly decrease in the number of eggs so that at birth, only a million remain. By puberty, that number is down to 300,000. Only a lucky 300 to 400 of these eggs ever actually ovulate over a lifetime.[1] The longer an egg lives, the higher the chance that changes can occur to the egg that will result either in its inability to be fertilized or an increased likelihood of producing a chromosomal abnormality such as Down syndrome.

There are ways to maximize the likelihood of pregnancy during any given cycle. You can take an average of a number of your cycles and determine the range of possibilities for ovulation and time intercourse around that. For example, if your cycles are such that you could ovulate anywhere between the 11th and 16th day of the cycle, plan to have intercourse every other day from day 10 to day 16.

Having intercourse every day, or multiple times a day as some of my overly zealous patients have done, is not necessary, as sperm can live for a couple of days. Also, having intercourse every day can decrease the amount of sperm per ejaculate, thus lowering your chance for conception on any particular day. This doesn't mean that if you had timed intercourse on Tuesday and just feel like having it on Wednesday, you shouldn't do so. Abstaining from sex for the first part of the month is also not recommended, as the number of dead sperm per ejaculation will be increased initially.

Basal body temperature charts, where you record your morning temperature every day immediately upon wakening and before having anything to eat or drink, can be used to gain information about your ovulation. The average morning basal temperature is low, less than 98.6 degrees Fahrenheit. When you ovulate, something called a corpus luteum is formed that produces progesterone to help support a developing embryo. Progesterone is a thermogenic agent, meaning it raises your core body temperature. When you ovulate, your core temperature will go up and remain up until

1. Cleveland Clinic, 2019.

your period starts. If conception occurs, the basal temperature will remain elevated throughout the pregnancy. There are a number of apps that take this information into account that you can use rather than manually taking your temperature every morning.

Note that the elevated temperature occurs after ovulation. Since conception is more likely to occur on or before ovulation, this method is more of a general guide to the window mentioned above than a method to pinpoint when to have intercourse. For that, you might want to use an over the counter ovulation predictor kit. This measures the luteinizing hormone (LH) surge that occurs one day before ovulation. Intercourse can be more precisely timed using these kits. However, they are expensive, and if your cycles are very irregular, the cost could add up over time.

Finding a Doctor

In the best of worlds, a woman wishing to become pregnant and her partner should consult her provider prior to trying to conceive. This is the perfect time to review their medical and family histories. At the very least, the issues that follow should be discussed.

If you do not have an obstetrician, this is a good time to find one. Your choice might depend upon which hospital you would like to deliver at. Medical staff offices are happy to provide you with lists of obstetricians who deliver at their hospital. If possible, make an appointment for a meet-and-greet to get a better idea of the practice.

Do you want a solo practitioner, or group of two or more physicians who work together, sharing patients and responsibilities? If you choose a group, you will have the opportunity to meet all of the physicians who might be there for your delivery but will not know which one will actually be there for your delivery, as the call schedule usually determines that. If you choose a solo practitioner, you will see the same person every visit, which can be quite comforting. However, he or she will likely share call with other physicians or laborists (obstetricians who work full-time at a hospital) because no doctor can be on call 24 hours a day, 365 days a year. Not only would this be impractical, it is dangerous. Thus, you may end up being delivered by someone you have never met. If it is important for you to have a close relationship with one or two individuals, choose the latter. If you are concerned about knowing the face of the person who is there during your labor and delivery, you may want to select the former option. The choice is yours. Above all, look for a person or group who has philosophies of care that align with yours.

Insurance

When searching for an OB/GYN, it's important to pay attention to whether the group or solo practitioner, and the hospital you will deliver at, takes your insurance. This is not a trivial concern these days. In 2018, the average cost for having a baby in the United States ranged from $5,000 to $11,000. If you have a Cesarean section, the price ranges from $7,000 to $14,500.[2] The price can vary tremendously depending upon where you live, with higher costs on the coasts and in major cities. High-risk pregnancies and birth complications can add additional amounts.

Your insurance coverage will determine how much of that total you are responsible for. If you have a Health Maintenance Organization (HMO), your provider has agreed to accept whatever the insurance company will pay, minus any deductible, for the entire pregnancy. If you have a Preferred Provider Organization (PPO), there may be many caveats: only two ultrasounds are allowed; lab tests might be covered, but only at the insurance company's lab of choice; and you must pay all deductibles before you receive any reimbursement.

Services at the hospital that are not covered by insurance can be a sticking point. For instance, if the hospital accepts your insurance but the anesthesiologist that puts in your epidural does not, you will be responsible for any overages on your epidural. You should know that "usual and customary" is the amount the insurance company is willing to pay, not the actual usual and customary fee charged in your area. Please do your research here. Your

---

2. Houston, 2019.

provider cannot know what your employer has agreed with your insurance company to cover.

If your provider does not accept your insurance, there will be a big gap between what you are billed and what you are reimbursed. It's the insurance company's way of pressing you to use their preferred providers. If the gap is large, or if you don't have maternity benefits at all, do not be afraid to speak with the billing department to see if you can work out a reduced fee or payment plan. Babies are expensive enough as it is. You do not want to get a surprise bill a couple of months later.

When To Stop Birth Control

If you are taking any form of hormonal birth control, it is recommended that you stop at least two cycles before trying to conceive. Use condoms or another form of birth control during this time, and don't forget to start taking your prenatal vitamins (more on that in the next section). If you accidentally get pregnant before the two months is up, don't worry. The old idea that the pill remains in your system for six months and can cause birth defects if conception occurs during that time is simply not based on fact.

The real reason for asking women to wait a couple of months is to give her and her provider an idea of what her cycles are like without birth control and thus, a better clue as to when she ovulates. This information, along with an early pregnancy test and ultrasound, can be helpful in determining the exact age of a baby. Many decisions are made later in pregnancy based on the gestational age, such as whether or not to give steroids to help mature a baby's lungs for early delivery, or whether or not to induce a pregnancy past the anticipated due date.

Many women today have been on birth control pills since they were in high school or college because of irregular cycles, heavy or painful periods, or simply for birth control. They have absolutely no idea what their cycles will be like off of the pill. Please do not be concerned if your periods are suddenly every 25 to 32 days instead of the predictable 28 days on the pill. That is artificial. I cannot tell you how many phone calls I've received from women trying to conceive who are worried that there may be something wrong because their cycles are no longer like clockwork. The human body is predictably unpredictable.

There are many women (and hopeful grandmothers) who are concerned that the length of time on the pill will affect their ability to ovulate again and conceive. When my patients express this concern, I often ask them to consider the following scenario: if you put a huge boulder in a rushing stream, the water runs around it. Years later, if you remove the boulder, the water immediately rushes in to cover the area. Your body is like this. It so badly wants to ovulate that you have to actively stop it from doing so, whether with a pill every single day, a vaginal ring such as the NuvaRing, or a progesterone shot every three months (Depo-Provera). When you stop taking these kinds of birth control, your body usually begins to ovulate almost immediately, just as it did before taking the pill.

Other forms of birth control do not necessarily stop ovulation. For example, implants, such as Nexplanon, do not always inhibit ovulation and IUDs containing progesterone or copper work locally in the uterus, cervix, and fallopian tubes to prevent pregnancy.

Prenatal Vitamins

It is important to start taking folic acid—0.4 mg a day—at least a month before pregnancy and during the first couple months of pregnancy. This will significantly reduce the risk of the fetus developing neural tube defects (abnormalities of the spinal cord and brain) such as spina bifida or meningomyelocele. Because the neural tube is completely formed by 10 weeks, the folic acid must be present at the beginning of pregnancy. All multivitamins in the United States, by law, must contain at least 0.4 mg of folic acid because many pregnancies are unintended. Some women, such as those with twins or on certain anti-seizure medications, will need to take more than 0.4 mg. This should be discussed with your provider.

There is a plethora of expensive prenatal vitamins on the market today. Truth be told, the supermarket brand is likely just as effective as the higher priced ones that contain DHA, fish oil, stool softeners, and other agents to make the pill more palatable. The American College of Obstetricians and Gynecologists simply recommends the folic acid as well as vitamin D and iron.[3]

Most prenatal vitamins contain iron. Because women have to make all of their baby's red blood cells plus two units of extra blood for themselves during pregnancy, it is likely that they will, at some point in the pregnancy, need additional iron. While iron might be necessary for your health and that of your baby, it does have its drawbacks: iron has a tendency to cause constipation. Pregnancy, especially the first trimester, does an excellent job of causing constipation as well. Stool softeners work by keeping more water in the gastrointestinal tract and making the stool softer. You can look for vitamins that contain stool softeners, keep your fluid intake high, and/ or eat more raw spinach or prunes.

DHA is a trendy addition to many vitamins these days. It is essential in human diets and is found in fish and some vegetable oils. Will your child be smarter or run faster or jump higher if he or she is provided with extra amounts of this nutrient in utero? Probably not, but it's a good thing to include in your diet. You can get it in your vitamins, or you can eat the allowed fish a few times a week.

Lifestyle

Your health concerns when you are preparing for pregnancy or are already carrying a baby differ in many ways from those of women at other times in their lives. The following section reviews a number of the issues that pregnant women or soon-to-be moms should consider.

Exercise

It's important that you stay active for the duration of your pregnancy. Aim to establish a moderate exercise plan consisting of aerobic activity at least

---

3. Committee Opinion, 2011.

three times a week and strength training at least two times a week. Do not overdo it, as it is important for you to be able to continue these activities throughout your pregnancy. Will being in shape make your labor shorter or less painful? Absolutely not. But your endurance and stamina will increase.

Internal Body Temperature

The use of saunas and hot tubs has the potential to raise the core body temperature. Temperature levels of 100.4 degrees Fahrenheit or higher, in general, have been associated with miscarriage and malformations.[4] Is there data to prove that doing so will result in miscarriage? Not that I am aware of, but it would seem prudent to either avoid these options or at least monitor your temperature while partaking in either activity. Bikram yoga, which is done in a room temperature of 105 degrees, rarely raises the core body temperature above 99 degrees.

Vaccinations and Viruses

Are your immunizations up to date? If not, please make certain they are. If you will be traveling to developing nations during your pregnancy, please look into vaccines that will be needed and whether or not they are "live." All live vaccines are contraindicated in pregnancy. Malaria prophylaxis is indicated at any point in pregnancy. Malaria and pregnancy absolutely do not do well together.

If you have small children or work or volunteer at a day care center or preschool, you should be tested for immunity to parvovirus B19. This virus, also known as fifth disease or slap disease, is relatively harmless in children but can cause serious problems for your baby, especially if you are exposed to it in the first trimester.

Also, you should check with the CDC if you are planning to travel to countries with Zika virus. Exposure of you or your partner both before and during pregnancy can affect your baby. Recommendations are constantly

---

4. Toby, 2018.

changing and being updated. You should check with your obstetrician, primary care provider, the CDC, and/or a travel clinic before international trips.

Pregnancy and influenza are a potentially bad combination for both the fetus and the mother. Fetuses do not do well with sustained maternal temperatures, and the immunocompromised state, or weakened immune system, of pregnant women predisposes them to complications they would not otherwise expect. Just like the elderly, those with respiratory illnesses, and those with HIV/AIDS or other weakened immune system states, pregnant women are much more likely to end up in the ICU on a respirator than otherwise healthy individuals if they get the flu. Please, if you are going to be pregnant during flu season, get your flu shot. It does not contain a live virus and has been demonstrated over the years to be perfectly safe for pregnant women to receive, even in the first trimester.

American College of Obstetricians and Gynecologists (ACOG) Recommendations

The following is a listing of the most recent ACOG recommendations taken from a 2018 article in Obstetrics and Gynecology.[5] The italicized text is taken directly from the article while the regular text is comprised of my own thoughts and research on the subject matter. You may find that you can now enjoy, guilt-free, an occasional glass of wine, a cup of coffee, and some sushi!

ACOG classifies its recommendations as level A, B, or C: [6]

- Level A recommendations are "based on good and consistent scientific evidence."

- Level B recommendations are "based on limited or inconsistent scientific evidence."

---

5. Fox, 2018.
6. The American College of Obstetricians and Gynecologists, 2018.

- Level C recommendations are "based primarily on consensus and expert opinion."

Alcohol

Although current data suggest that consumption of small amounts of alcohol during pregnancy (less than seven to nine drinks/wk) does not appear to be harmful to the fetus, the exact threshold between safe and unsafe, if it exists, is unknown. (Level B)

Alcohol should be avoided in pregnancy (Level C)

Regular and heavy use of alcohol during pregnancy, especially in the third trimester when fetal brain growth is at its greatest, can result in a devastating condition associated with mental retardation and behavioral disorders. Will an occasional glass of wine result in fetal alcohol syndrome? No. Will being drunk at your best friend's wedding the night you conceive result in fetal alcohol syndrome? No. The problem is that there is a continuum between occasional or recreational alcohol consumption and excessive amounts that can lead to fetal harm. No one can tell you what the crossover point is, so, if you wish to drink during pregnancy, please limit consumption to an occasional glass of wine. And, for your own safety, do not do so in public if you are clearly pregnant because there are crusaders out there who will definitely bring this risk to your attention, sometimes not too subtly.

Artificial Sweeteners

Artificial sweeteners can be used in pregnancy.

Data regarding saccharin are conflicting. Low (typical) consumption is likely safe. (Level B)

A number of reports have surfaced over the years suggesting that artificial sweeteners have been linked to the development of various cancers, but these have not been substantiated. If you wish to avoid excessive calorie intake to maintain a healthy weight, feel free to consume moderate amounts of these substances.

Caffeine

Low-to-moderate caffeine intake in pregnancy does not appear to be associated with any adverse outcomes.

Pregnant women may have caffeine but should probably limit it to less than 300 milligrams per day ([a] typical 8-ounce cup of brewed coffee has approximately 130 mg of caffeine. An 8-ounce cup of tea or 12-ounce soda has approximately 50 mg of caffeine), but exact amounts vary based on the specific beverage or food. (Level B)

Caffeine crosses the placenta and can be found in amniotic fluid and fetal blood. The fetus metabolizes the caffeine that it is exposed to very slowly, so even low maternal consumption can lead to prolonged fetal exposure. In addition, the mother's ability to process, or break down, caffeine decreases significantly as pregnancy progresses.

Most studies demonstrate no effect of caffeine on the fetus at levels less than 300 mg per day. Caffeine has been "associated" in various studies in the past with fertility problems, increased miscarriage rates, congenital abnormalities, pregnancy complications that are mostly related to blood pressure elevation, and some behavioral problems in children. However, after adjusting for lifestyle factors such as fertility, maternal age, and smoking and alcohol consumption, very little evidence exists to support detrimental effects of caffeine on fertility and/or pregnancy in normally consumed amounts.[7]

Fish Consumption

Pregnant women should try to consume two to three servings per week of fish with a high DHA (Docosahexaenoic acid, an essential poly-

---

7. Committee Opinion, 2010.

unsaturated fatty acid required for brain and eye growth) *and low mercury content.* (Level A)

For women who do not achieve this, it is unknown whether DHA or n-3 pufa (polyunsaturated omega-3 fatty acid) *supplementation is beneficial, but they are unlikely to be harmful.* (Level B)[8]

Raw or Undercooked Fish

In line with current recommendations, pregnant women should generally avoid undercooked fish. However, sushi that was prepared in a clean and reputable establishment is unlikely to pose a risk to the pregnancy. (Level B)

Methylmecury can damage developing neural systems. The more methylmecury that accumulates and the longer the exposure time, the more severe the risk for damage to the fetus will be. The main source of methylmercury in fish comes from industrial pollution contained in rain, snow, and water run-off. As the water—and the pollution within it—enters streams, oceans, rivers, and lakes, it is transformed into mercury by bacteria. Larger and older fish accumulate more mercury, thus making them riskier for pregnant women to consume. King mackerel, shark, swordfish, and tilefish should be avoided completely, while limited amounts (6 ounces or less a week) of bluefish, grouper, orange or red roughy, marlin, and fresh tuna can be safely consumed.

"Light" tuna is processed from smaller species of tuna and has decreased concentrations of mercury as compared with white (albacore) or tuna steaks and fillets, which should be limited to 6 ounces per week. Catfish, clams, cod, flounder, sole, haddock, herring, ocean perch, rainbow trout, oyster, farmed salmon, wild salmon, scallops, shrimp, tilapia, and farmed trout are all safe for consumption at any level.

---

8. life'sDHA, 2018.

It should be noted that cooking a fish that is high in mercury does not reduce the level or harm posed to the developing fetus.[9]

Other Foods To Avoid (Level B)

Pregnant women should avoid raw and undercooked meat.

Pregnant women should wash vegetables and fruit before eating them.

Pregnant women should avoid unpasteurized dairy products.

Unheated deli meats could also potentially increase the risk of listeria, but the risk in recent years is uncertain.

Pregnant women should avoid foods that are being recalled for possible listeria contamination.

The FDA advises pregnant women, the elderly, and those with weakened immune systems to avoid the use of unpasteurized cheeses or those that have been aged less than 60 days. This is to avoid the risk of exposure to a bacterium called *Listeria monocytogenes*, which causes listeriosis.

Pasteurized cheeses or those aged over 60 days are generally considered safe if they are kept under constant refrigeration. Since 1949, the U.S. government has forbidden the commercial sale of cheeses made from unpasteurized milk unless aged at least 60 days. After 60 days, the acids and salts in raw milk cheese naturally prevent listeria as well as salmonella and E. coli growth. Thus, if a woman consumes commercial cheeses purchased in the U.S., even if they are soft cheeses, she is, in fact, at little to no risk. The danger lies with cheeses sold in places like farmer's markets or the trendy new farm-to-table restaurants that are made from raw milk to, in theory, preserve their flavor and healthful advantages. Generally, though, if raw milk cheeses are aged for 60 days or more, they too may be consumed safely. The only unpasteurized cheese I was able to find in Whole Foods after an extensive search was Parmesan, but it had been aged for 24 months.[10]

---

9. U.S. Food and Drug Administration, 2019.
10. U.S. Food and Drug Administration, 2017.

Smoking, Nicotine, and Vaping

Women should not smoke cigarettes during pregnancy. If they are unable to quit entirely, they should reduce it as much as possible.

Nicotine replacement (with patches or gum) is appropriate as part of a smoking cessation strategy. (Level B)

Cigarette smoking is an absolute "no-no" for anyone who may be pregnant. All sorts of harms—including miscarriage, hypertensive disorders such as preeclampsia, and eclampsia, and fetal growth restriction—have been traced to the use of tobacco products. If you have trouble quitting, try using a patch instead. Although it contains nicotine, at least it does not contain the noxious gases associated with smoking cigarettes. No data exist for the effects of vaping while pregnant on a fetus, but until proven otherwise, that habit should be avoided during pregnancy as well.

Marijuana Use

Marijuana use in not known to be associated with any adverse outcomes in pregnancy. (Level C)

However, data regarding long-term neurodevelopmental outcomes are lacking: therefore, marijuana use is currently not recommended in pregnancy.

Marijuana is the colloquial term for the buds, leaves, and stems of the cannabis plant that is most often smoked, although it can be consumed by other methods. Marijuana has significant levels of tetrahydrocannabinol (THC), the primary psychoactive chemical present within the drug. Will THC cause birth defects? Probably not. Is there a drug equivalent to fetal alcohol syndrome? Not that is known. However, you should not consume something while you are pregnant that you would not give to or do around your baby after he or she is born.

Kitty Litter

If you have a cat, you may be exposed to the Toxoplasma gondii parasite in the litter. This is a common parasite that causes Toxoplasmosis. While you are actually more likely to be exposed from unwashed vegetables, you should probably avoid changing litter boxes, especially in the third trimester, if you can. If you must change the litter, consider wearing a mask and gloves when you do so. The same holds true if you garden or play in outdoor sandboxes with your niece or nephew during pregnancy, as these can become large outdoor litter boxes.

Routine screening of all pregnant women is not recommended in the U.S. but monthly or every three-month testing is performed in parts of Europe, most strictly in France. The risk of fetal infection increases with advancing pregnancy. Owning a cat is only weakly associated with acute infection because cats only excrete the eggs for a three-week period in their lifetime. Fresh cat feces are not infectious.[11,12]

Peanuts

A 2008 statement by the American Academy of Pediatrics concluded that there is not sufficient evidence to recommend that a woman whose child is at risk for allergic disorders (at least one first-degree relative with documented allergic disease) avoid allergenic foods such as peanuts, eggs, and milk during pregnancy or lactation for the purpose of preventing allergic diseases in their children. This recommendation came in April 2019 after a review of numerous studies suggesting these benefits revealed significant flaws in study design. So, enjoy peanuts, milk, and eggs during your pregnancy; they will not cause harm to your baby.[13]

11. Committee Opinion, 2016.
12. Gilbert and Petersen, 2018.
13. Greer, Sicherer and Burks, 2008.

Genetics and Family History

Prior to your visit with your OB, please check with family members about any history of congenital or genetic abnormalities in your family. You would be surprised by how many family secrets may be lurking out there. Frequent miscarriages can also be a clue. If you and your partner have not had genetic testing, this is the time to do so. There are a number of recessive genetic disorders such as cystic fibrosis, sickle cell anemia, Thalassemia, Tay Sachs, Canavan's, Gaucher's, and familial dysautonomia that are more prevalent in certain ethnic groups, such as those of Jewish, African, and Mediterranean descent. With any recessive disorder, if both parents carry the trait, there is a 25 percent chance that their baby will inherit a devastating disorder. Having this information before pregnancy can allow for calm and measured evaluation of both individuals, along with genetic counseling.

If you are 35 years of age or over, please discuss with your doctor the risks of "advanced maternal age," including higher rates of chromosomal abnormalities and medical complications during pregnancy. Fortunately, screening for chromosomal abnormalities can now be done with a blood test at 10 weeks. The even better news is that you can learn the gender of your baby with that test if you are so inclined. Be prepared to have more monitoring, including ultrasounds, if you are older, and know that your physician may recommend that you be induced on or before your due date to reduce risk to your baby if you are 40 or older.

Medications

Various medications can affect fetal growth and development. To help providers and women determine which drugs are safe for use in pregnancy and which are not, the Federal Drug Administration in 1979, established safety risk categories for prescription drug use during pregnancy labeled A, B, C, D, or X. However, because of patient and provider complaints that the system was an overly simplistic grading system, a new one was rolled out in 2015 and completed in 2018. The lettered categories were replaced with narratives that include exposure registries, risk summaries, clinical considerations, and data. While more informative, in general, there are no definitive "yes" or "no" answers. Individuals, instead, are required to interpret the information on a case-by-case basis.

For the sake of simplicity, I will describe the recommendations based on the old categories.[14,15]

Category A (aka "safe") drugs are those that can be taken with minimal to no concern because according to the FDA, "adequate and well-controlled studies have failed to demonstrate a risk to the fetus in the first trimester of pregnancy (and there is no evidence of risk in later trimesters)." This translates to either a note from God saying the drug is safe or water from a pure spring in the remote Himalayas.

Category B (aka "probably safe") medications are those that have been used for years in pregnant women. The FDA has found that "animal reproduction studies have failed to demonstrate a risk to the fetus and there are no adequate and well-controlled studies in pregnant women OR animal studies have shown an adverse effect, but adequate and well-controlled studies in pregnant women have failed to demonstrate a risk to the fetus in any trimester." Most over-the-counter medications fall into this category. Basically, if you can get it without a prescription, it's probably safe for you to consume while pregnant.

Please note that products such as NSAIDs (nonsteroidal anti-inflammatory drugs) such as aspirin, Motrin, or ibuprofen, while safe in terms of the baby, do cause the blood to "thin." As such, they are not recommended in the first trimester when the risk for bleeding from miscarriage is high. All of them can lead to something called a patent ductus arteriosus that results in abnormal blood flow between two of the major arteries connected to the heart at delivery, which can be harmful to newborns. Thus, these agents are not recommended in the third trimester. If you pull a muscle and want to

---

14. Federal Register, 2008.
15. U.S. Food and Drug Administration, 2018.

take effective medication, you might want to do so in the second trimester when these drugs are safe to take.

Category C (aka "some potential problems but benefit may outweigh risk") drugs are labeled as such because "animal reproduction studies have shown an adverse effect on the fetus and there are no adequate and well-controlled studies in humans, but potential benefits may warrant use of the drug in pregnant women despite potential risks." Many of the medications used to treat blood pressure, asthma, depression, and other common conditions fall into this category. It is important to discuss these with your provider in advance of becoming pregnant.

Category D (aka "do not use this drug unless absolutely necessary") drugs have "positive evidence of human fetal risk based on adverse reaction data from investigational or marketing experience or studies in humans, but potential benefits may warrant use of the drug in pregnant women despite potential risks." Some anti-seizure medications fall into this category.

Category X (aka "do not use") medications are those in which "studies in animals or humans have demonstrated fetal abnormalities and/or there is positive evidence of human fetal risk based on adverse reaction data from investigational or marketing experience, and the risks involved in use of the drug in pregnant women clearly outweigh potential benefits." An example would be medications to lower cholesterol.

Not too infrequently, women will recall at their first visit that they had a febrile illness or took medications or used drugs or alcohol before they knew they were pregnant. There is no specific blood test to determine if these substances affected your baby. However, if you had a viral illness, a test called the Torch (Toxoplasmosis, Other, Rubella, Cytomegalovirus, Herpes) Titer can be drawn to determine if there has been recent exposure to these viruses. Sonograms are helpful to determine if the baby is structurally normal and is growing appropriately. While these tests cannot guarantee a healthy baby, negative results can be very reassuring.

Medical Illnesses

Many medical illnesses can and do have an effect on pregnancy and vice versa. If, for example, you have a thyroid disorder, you will need to monitor your thyroid stimulating hormone (TSH) levels throughout the pregnancy, as adjustments may need to be made to your dosage to prevent miscarriage or potential mental retardation for your baby.

Diabetes

If you have or develop diabetes during your pregnancy, your sugar levels will need to be monitored closely to avoid complications with the fetus. Such complications could include the fetus being large for gestational age (LGA), which can result in the need for a cesarean delivery or worse, birth trauma resulting in lifetime limitations for your baby. Elevated maternal blood sugar levels during labor can cause your baby to have low blood sugars at birth, which could require treatment with intravenous glucose after delivery. Sustained elevated blood sugars prior to and during the first trimester can result in miscarriage or birth defects.

High Blood Pressure

High blood pressure can result in fetal growth restriction or lead to the development of conditions such as preeclampsia and eclampsia, which I will elaborate on later.

Pelvic Issues

A history of endometriosis or pelvic infection might have resulted in damage to your fallopian tubes. This could make it difficult for you to become pregnant and increases the risk for an ectopic pregnancy (a pregnancy outside of the uterine cavity, which cannot survive, and can result in catastrophic bleeding).

Sexually Transmitted Diseases

Do you have a history of genital herpes? If so, and if you get an infection around the time of birth, this virus can be passed on to your baby and result in devastating neurologic consequences. Prophylactic (preventive) doses of Valtrex starting at the 36th week of pregnancy are recommended by the American College of Obstetricians and Gynecologists to reduce the likelihood of transmitting the virus to babies who are delivered vaginally.[16]

HIV/AIDS can be passed on to your baby. If you know you are infected or it is determined that you have it by blood tests during the pregnancy that you are, you will be referred to a specialist to treat you in order to decrease the risk of transmission to your baby.

Untreated gonorrhea and chlamydia can result in preterm delivery, low birth weight, and newborn eye infections. Syphilis infection can result in something called congenital syphilis and has been linked to prematurity, stillbirths, and developmental abnormalities. You will be tested for these sexually transmitted infections at the beginning and end of your pregnancy and treated as indicated. In some states, you will also be tested for some of these infections in the second trimester.

The above is not to be considered an exhaustive list of disorders that can lead to problems for you or you baby. I just wanted to provide a general overview of the problems that I most often see. Please use the time before you conceive, if possible, to review your and your family's medical history in detail with your provider.

---

16. Committee Opinion, 2007.

When to Seek Help

If your ovulations or menstrual cycles are not regular, for instance, if you have polycystic ovarian syndrome (PCOS), you might want to speak with your physician early in the course of trying to conceive. There are medications to induce ovulation "on command" that are generally quite safe when used appropriately.

If you have a history of pelvic infection or endometriosis and either don't get pregnant in a year with untimed intercourse or after three or four cycles of timed intercourse, you might wish to consult a fertility specialist. So many advancements have been made in the field in recent years that this once devastating problem becomes a minor bump in the road for many. (That is, if you consider the time, money, hormones, etc. required for in vitro fertilization just a "bump.") But there truly is reason to be positive about your chances for conception nowadays.

Age 35 has often been looked upon as the turning point for fertility. This is not a magic age at which you suddenly become infertile, but it is numerically the place where the slope of the line starts to increase, with each successive year becoming more difficult to conceive. It is also the time when the risk for chromosomal abnormalities becomes more marked. The risk for having a baby with Down syndrome from age 20 to 24 is 1/1,400. At 35 years old, the risk is 1/350. At 40, the risk is 1/100 with the risk of any chromosomal abnormality reaching 1/63.[17] These are sobering statistics, indeed.

---

17. Hook, Cross and Schreinemachers, 1983.

Frequency of Down Syndrome
Per Maternal Age

Age (years)	Frequency of Fetuses with Down Syndrome to Normal Fetuses at 16 weeks of pregnancy	Frequency of Live Births of Babies with Down Syndrome to Normal Births
15–19	—	1 / 1,250
20–24	—	1 / 1,400
25–29	—	1 / 1,100
30–31	—	1 / 900
32	—	1 / 750
33	1 / 420	1 / 625
34	1 / 325	1 / 500
35	1 / 250	1 / 350
36	1 / 200	1 / 275
37	1 / 150	1 / 225
38	1 / 120	1 / 175
39	1 / 100	1 / 140
40	1 / 75	1 / 100
41	1 / 60	1 / 85
42	1 / 45	1 / 65
43	1 / 35	1 / 50
44	1 / 30	1 / 40
45 and older	1 / 20	1 / 25

The numbers are approximated and rounded.
Using this data, geneticists have set the number separating low-risk from high-risk at 1 / 250.

Why is there a difference in frequencies between 16 weeks and time of birth? Because of the spontaneous miscarriages of pregnancies with Down syndrome between these times.

For more information on risks of more detailed situations (such as translocation or mothers who have had previous babies with Down syndrome, see Dr. Benke's essay on Risk and Recurrence of Down syndrome.

Reference for the above table: Hook EB. JAMA 249:2034-2038, 1983.

However, many women can, and do, conceive without a problem in their mid-to-late 30s. The closer to 40 a woman gets, the lower her chances for conception and the higher her risk for miscarriage. Spontaneous conception from 40 to 42 does occur, but assisted reproductive technology becomes more common in this age group. Over age 42, the likelihood of requiring donor eggs becomes significant.

We have all heard about movie stars and other well-known women who have had babies in their mid-to-late 40s. Unfortunately, knowing this, some women put off trying for pregnancy based on what seems to be an easily doable thing. Be advised that it is possible to conceive, but you must be willing to consider using donor eggs, something that not everyone is either interested in or able to afford, unless you froze your eggs when you were in your early 30s.

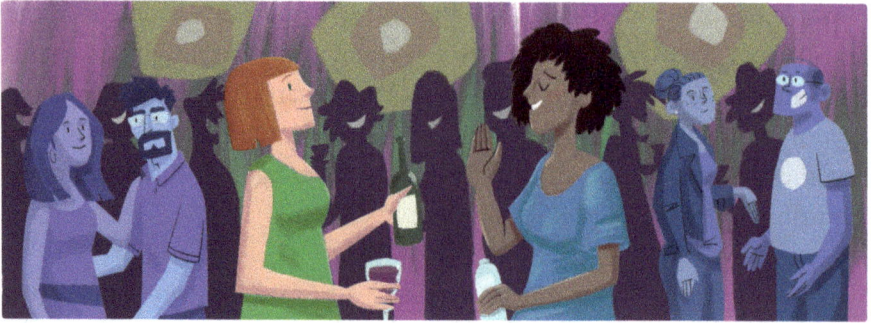
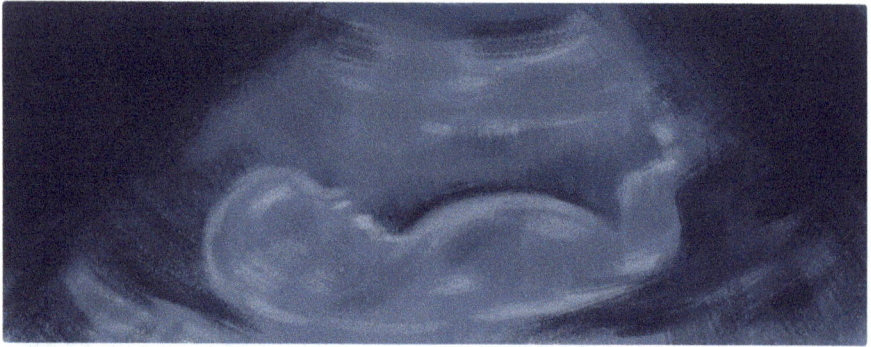
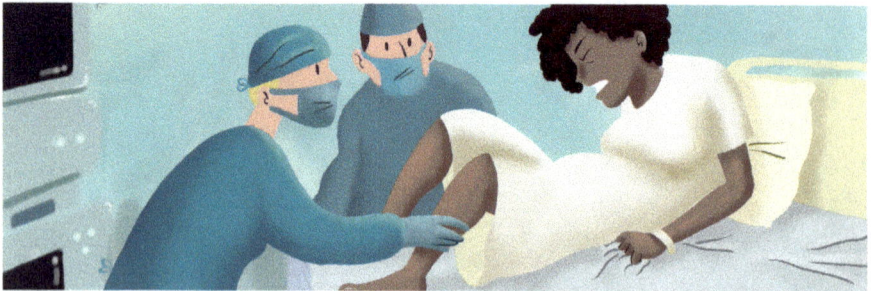
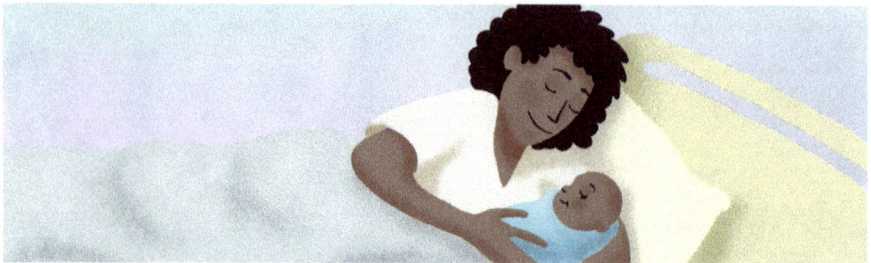

Part Two

Pregnancy Considerations

There are many references and textbooks out there that go into very detailed descriptions of the numerous tests, the baby's size at different times, and potential complications during the various stages of pregnancy. It is not my desire to replicate those well-researched compendiums. Rather, in this section about pregnancy and labor and delivery, I intend to discuss what I see as the more salient issues with an emphasis on those areas I have found to be more frequently of concern to my patients instead of bogging you down with a great deal of detail.

First Trimester

Congratulations! It's the day you expected your period, you take a pregnancy test, and it's positive. You take another one, and it's positive too. The next morning you take one, okay two, more. They are all positive. What should you do?

First, arrange to have a blood pregnancy test taken by your doctor. This will not only confirm your home tests, it will also give an actual value for your human chorionic gonadotropin (HCG), or pregnancy hormone level. This number will help your doctor determine if the pregnancy is a healthy one. Levels that are too low can mean possible miscarriage or ectopic pregnancy (a pregnancy outside the uterus) or incorrect conception dates, while levels that are too high could mean you are pregnant with more than one baby or that you miscalculated the conception dates, i.e. you are more or less pregnant than you thought you were.

A point of confusion for many here is that they are told they are six weeks pregnant at their first visit when they know they ovulated four weeks ago. This is because obstetrical dating is based on the first day of the last menstrual period as opposed to embryologic dating, which is based on the date of conceptions, i.e. how old the fetus actually is. Since the majority of women can recall the first day of their last menstrual period and very few can tell you when they actually ovulated or conceived, obstetricians base their "due date" on the last menstrual period. Basically, you are not pregnant the first two weeks of your pregnancy, the easiest time of gestation.

Obstetrical Myths
First Babies Are Always Late

Naegele's rule for determining a due date was established in 1806 and was based on 28-day cycles and a 280-day average pregnancy. The estimated date of delivery (EDD) or "due date" was determined by counting backwards three months from the last menstrual period and adding seven days.[18] There was no proviso for first or subsequent babies.

The Talmud places the length of pregnancy at 271-273 days (from the seventh, or last, day of the menstrual cycle, rather than from the first day.) "A woman becomes pregnant and gives birth after 271 to 273 days." The Hebrew word for pregnancy is 271 (Niddah 38).[19] Again, there is no proviso for first or subsequent babies.

---

18. Baskett and Nagele, 2000.
19. The Jewish Agency For Israel, 2005.

In doing research for a presentation a few years ago, I was able to find many articles that quoted many other articles as sources for the assertion that first pregnancies are often late. The problem is, there were very few actual studies. One article that is often referred to was from 1990 by a Harvard professor named Mittendorf.[20] His conclusion was that first-time mothers delivered late by an average of eight days. Unfortunately, this was based on data from just one study of only a few hundred women in private practices and included only 31 women in their first pregnancy. Based on this, the authors recommended counting back three months from the first day of the last menstrual period and adding 15 days for primips (those who are pregnant for the first time) and 10 days for multips (those who have had at least one delivery).

The National Survey of Family Growth did a study with more subjects in 2002. A total of 7,643 women were surveyed. Findings were that first babies were born 0.078 weeks later, or 13 hours, which is not statistically significant.[21]

All of this is to say that if you were given a "due date" based on a known last menstrual period with regular cycles and/or a first trimester ultrasound, you should count on that. 80 percent of babies are born within two weeks of this date, even those conceived with IVF, when the actual conception date is known exactly. Babies are done when they are done.

The next step is to make an appointment for your first visit, which may be just to perform an ultrasound to confirm viability or to discuss genetic testing and review your medical history. If this is not your first pregnancy, please be prepared to provide information about previous pregnancies, miscarriages, medical and obstetrical complications, and whether you had vaginal or cesarean deliveries.

---

20. Mittendorf, Williams, Berkey, and Cotter, 1990.
21. Centers for Disease Control and Prevention, 2019.

If you have had one or two first-trimester terminations (abortions) in the past, there should not be an effect on your current pregnancy. If you have had three or more terminations or have had a second-trimester termination, you may be at risk for developing something called an incompetent cervix that can result in second trimester loss. You will also be at risk for this if you have had a Loop Electrical Excision Procedure (LEEP) or cone biopsy, which are procedures done to remove precancerous changes from your cervix. You should expect to have frequent ultrasounds in order to monitor your cervix if this is the case.

You will be asked about your family history and that of your partner, as well as your and your partner's ethnicity. This is because there are many genetic abnormalities that are familial or more prevalent in various ethnic groups that can affect the health of your baby. If you have not already had genetic testing, this is the time to do so.

You will also be asked if you own a cat, have or are around preschool children on a regular basis, and whether or not you have herpes. Please see the section on Preconception Considerations for more details.

Medical Concerns

Signs and Symptoms

Fatigue is quite common during the first trimester. You may sleep 10 hours on the weekend, get up and have breakfast, and then feel the need to take a nap because of all the energy you just expended. This is normal and will pass.

I distinctly remember a specific instance in the first trimester of my first pregnancy when I pulled into my driveway and looked at the three steps leading to the walkway and the additional step up to the porch and determined that I simply could not do it. Instead, I took a 10-minute nap before negotiating the trek.

During your first pregnancy, your partner will likely dote on you and try to ease your everyday tasks. Be prepared for a different situation during your second or third pregnancies when you have a toddler or another older child. Your partner will likely already be overwhelmed as well and will be unable to dote quite as much; enjoy the attention while you can during the first one.

Mood swings are common during this time — and during the remainder of the pregnancy. Hormones are raging, and your body is going through many changes. Try to remember this when things that otherwise wouldn't irritate you make you crazy. If you suffer from depression, anxiety or other mood disorders, this would not be a good time to stop necessary, safe medications.

Nausea and Nutrition

Nausea and vomiting are the most common signs of early pregnancy, a rite of passage, so to speak. For most women, it is simply a bother and a sign that the pregnancy is progressing well. For others, it can progress to the point of dehydration and, rarely, hospital admission for IV hydration and nutrition. If you are able to hold food and liquids down and are not losing weight — any loss over five pounds requires evaluation — then providers feel sorry for you but are not worried about you.

Balanced nutrition is not the goal if you have significant nausea. Whatever makes you not what to throw up is what you should eat or drink. If particular healthy foods make you throw up, don't eat them. Most women start pregnancy in a healthy enough state that malnutrition is not a likely possibility. So, if cookies and chips make you feel good, eat cookies and chips, although, hopefully, something a bit more substantial will do the trick.

To avoid dehydration and/or weight loss, the following are recommended:

- Small, frequent meals

- Avoidance of spicy and greasy foods and strong odors

- Wet to dry regimen with alteration of solid and fluid intake

- Vitamin B6 with or without the antihistamine Unisom

- Ginger tea

- Lemon drops

- Sea bands (acupressure wristbands)

Medications are available if these options do not work.

Diet and Weight Gain

The American College of Obstetricians and Gynecologists currently recommends increasing your caloric intake by 350 to 450 calories a day depending on your pre-pregnancy Body Mass Index (BMI). Overweight and/or "vertically challenged" individuals should aim for lower numbers.[22] Thin and/or tall women can aim for higher levels. Average-weight individuals should aim for a total gain of about 25 to 35 pounds.[23]

Most of this weight will be gained in the second and third trimesters, although some individuals will put on a lot of weight in the first trimester because they find that eating is the only thing that keeps them from throwing up. Others may either lose a bit of weight or not gain much at all in the first trimester because of their nausea and vomiting. It all tends to work out in the end.

While this may sound like a lot, getting the extra protein and dairy required for a healthy pregnancy can account for almost all of those extra calories. The old adage of eating for two, if followed, may well result in you looking like two! Your baby really does not need that brownie or those cupcakes; you may want them, but the baby definitely does not need them.

---

22. Fox, 2018.
23. Committee Opinion, 2013.

If you eat a full breakfast and then a midmorning snack "for the baby," and a full lunch and a mid-afternoon snack "for the baby," followed by a full dinner and an evening snack for you, you will likely increase your caloric intake by 600 or 700 calories, which will result in far more than the recommended weight gain. If you are under 30, this weight may fall off after the pregnancy. If you are over 30, it will sit there, look at you, and say, "What?!"

Frequent small feedings to avoid periods of low blood sugar are a good idea. A snack can be a piece of cheese and part of an apple, a low-fat yogurt, or a handful of nuts. Serving size is important here. Remember that good-for-you foods have calories too.

The majority of women will need to either increase their intake of dairy products and/or take supplements, as pregnant women require 1,000 mg of calcium a day (three or more servings of dairy products or calcium-fortified almond or soy milk a day).[24]

Most women will also need iron supplementation because, during their pregnancy, they must make all of their baby's red blood cells, as well as two units of extra red blood for themselves. Unless you eat large amounts of red meat, this is difficult to do on your own, and you should take iron supplements. Please make sure not to take the iron supplement at the same time as your calcium supplements, as they will bind to each other and then pass through the digestive tract unabsorbed. Either take these supplements at different times or consume them with meals to decrease the risk of their not being absorbed.

Avoid eating undercooked or uncooked meat, fish, or poultry. See the section on Fish Consumption in Chapter 1 for a more in-depth explanation. Despite this warning, sushi is now considered acceptable to consume by the American College of Obstetricians as long as it is fresh. I can't imagine a sushi lover eating anything but fresh sushi, but that's the recommendation.[25]

---

24. [22] Fox, 2018.
25. [22] Fox, 2018.

Swordfish, shark, mackerel, and tilefish can contain excessive levels of mercury, which can be harmful to a fetus. Avoid these species of fish during pregnancy. Unpasteurized cheeses or those aged less than 60 days should also be avoided. This is an FDA requirement for sale in stores, so you should be fine. If you eat cheeses from farmer's markets or trendy farm-to-table restaurants, they may be made from unpasteurized milk. I elaborate on this issue in Chapter 1.

Do try to include up to 12 ounces a week of fish in your diet — other than the ones mentioned above — as they are an excellent low-fat source of protein and DHA. If you are a vegetarian, you will need to focus on getting sufficient complete proteins in your diet. Dairy products can provide some of the needed additional protein, but if you are a vegan, you will need to work harder to get that protein.[26]

Exercise

The American College of Obstetricians and Gynecologists, in response to many requests from women, used to offer a target heart rate not to be exceeded during exercise while pregnant. Since so many variables affect that rate, such as the woman's level of fitness before pregnancy, a specific number is no longer given. Instead, women are encouraged to exercise at a moderate intensity or a level at which they can still easily carry on a conversation.

For heretofore couch potatoes, that may mean a brisk walk with your partner in the evenings. For those individuals who regularly exercised before getting pregnant, that may mean running three miles instead of five or running your previous distance over a longer period of time. You should be able to breathe normally and have a normal heart rate within five minutes or so of stopping. If you become fatigued, or if you develop contractions, stop immediately. Do less activity the next time you exercise or take longer to do it.

26. life'sDHA, 2018.

Refrain from performing exercises that require protective equipment for the simple reason that if you could reasonably expect risk of bodily harm when not pregnant, you should avoid that activity while pregnant. There should be no downhill skiing, roller blading, or skydiving. Think twice about cycling outside, especially on busy streets where drivers may feel compelled to aim at you. Racquetball and squash could result in injury from the hard, fast-moving ball and should probably be avoided. Tennis should be fine. (If you are bad enough at it that you are likely to be hit by the ball, you are likely not going to try that during pregnancy anyway.)

Genetic Testing

In the not-too-distant past, the only option a woman had to determine if her baby had a chromosomal abnormality, such as Down syndrome, was to undergo invasive genetic testing. Initially, the only option was amniocentesis, a test performed in the 16th week of pregnancy that involves inserting a needle under ultrasonic guidance into the amniotic sac to obtain fluid containing fetal cells. The chromosomes are then evaluated to determine if there are any abnormalities. Specific tests for known genetic disorders can also be done if there is a personal or family history that increases the likelihood of a specific disorder.

The problem with this form of testing is that it can't be done before 16 weeks, as there is generally not enough amniotic fluid available for testing before that time. It can take up to two weeks to get the results. Then, if an abnormality is found and termination is desired, a second trimester procedure is required. There is also a small—less than 1 percent—risk of miscarriage as a result of the procedure, even if done correctly.

Chorionic villi sampling (CVS) was developed in the 1980s. This test, which samples cells destined to develop into placental tissue, can be done in the first trimester. The risk for miscarriage may be a bit higher than for amniocentesis but is still very low, and termination, if desired, can then be performed at the end of the first trimester.

Fortunately, due to the ability to analyze cell-free fetal DNA in the maternal blood stream, these invasive tests are performed far less frequently today. Instead, at 10 weeks of pregnancy, a noninvasive pregnancy test (NIPT) can be drawn and analyzed for chromosomal and, if requested, various genetic abnormalities. The results are generally available in one to two weeks, depending on how much fetal DNA is present. The test will also determine if the fetus has a Y chromosome. If so, it's a boy. If a Y chromosome is not present, it's a girl.

Obstetrical Myths
Gender Determination

This is becoming a moot point today with the availability of tests for cell-free fetal DNA in the maternal circulation so that a couple can have blood drawn in week 10 of pregnancy to determine the gender. However, playing the guessing game can still be fun. Following are some of the more popular theories, the first seven of which I became aware of at a baby shower for a friend of mine a number of years ago.

- If you dangle a needle, pin, or wedding ring over the reclining mother's belly, it will swing like a pendulum if the baby is a boy and in a circular motion if it is a girl.

- If the baby's father gains weight, the baby is a boy.

- If the mother carries low and narrow, she will have a boy. If the mother carries high and wide she will have a girl.

- If quickening occurs early, the baby is a boy. If it occurs late, the baby is a girl.

- If the mother's left breast is larger than her right, the baby is a girl.

- If the linea negra (dark line down the center of the abdomen in pregnancy) extends only to the umbilicus (navel), then the baby is a girl. If it extends to the xyphoid (lower part of the sternum), it is a boy.

- If a pregnant woman urinates over Drano (1980s recipe), the solution will turn brown if the baby is a girl and green-blue if it is a boy.

- In Jewish tradition, the sex of the baby is determined at conception. "If a woman gives forth her seed first and bears a male child," the child will be a boy. "If a man gives forth his seed first and bears a girl," the child will be a girl.[27]

- If the heart rate is slow (less than 140 beats per minute), the baby is a boy. If the heart rate is fast (greater than 140 beats per minute), the baby is a girl.

- The Walter Reed "Test": The heart rate of babies on admission was recorded and a coin was flipped. The coin flip was as predictive of the gender as was the heart rate. (This was done unscientifically in my internship year.)

- An Egyptian papyrus from 1350 described a test wherein a potentially pregnant woman would urinate on wheat and barley seeds over several days. If the barley grew, the child was a male. If the wheat grew, it was a female. If neither grew, she was not pregnant. Testing of this theory in 1963 found that 70 percent of the time, the urine of pregnant women resulted in growth; urine from non-pregnant women and men did not.[28]

- The Chinese Lunar Calendar chart shows up on many websites for determining fetal gender. In theory, it was created some 700 years ago. The chart is supposed to have been discovered in a royal tomb in Beijing. Accuracy is quoted as anywhere from 75 percent to 90 percent and is based on the age and month of conception. Even results designate a boy and odd results designate a girl. According to this Chinese Lunar Calendar, which I did on an online site, my son is a girl and my daughter is a boy!

---

27. JEWNIVERSE, 2016.
28. Office of NIH History, 2003.

Most insurance companies will cover this test for women aged 35 and over because of their higher risk for chromosomal abnormalities. However, if you are under 35, many insurance companies do not yet cover the test (although this is changing rapidly), which can cost a few hundred dollars. Another option is an Ultra-Screen blood test at 10 weeks that is combined with a specialized ultrasound at 11-12 weeks to give you recalculated odds as to whether or not your baby has Down syndrome or Trisomy 13 or 18, by far the most common chromosomal abnormalities. If the risk is high, cell-free fetal DNA testing will then be offered and covered by insurance. If these results are also abnormal, amniocentesis will be offered to confirm. A pregnancy should never be terminated based on blood tests alone because false positives — meaning the test suggests an abnormality that does not exist — do occur, although the numbers are very low. Unfortunately, false negatives, which suggest the fetus is normal when it is not, also occur.

These tests must be done at specific times during the first part of the pregnancy. It is important to get the timing correct or the window of opportunity may be missed. Please note that normal test results do not guarantee a baby born without problems, but normal test results usually indicate that the chances of having a baby with a genetic disorder are low.

Advanced Maternal Age

For various understandable reasons, many women do not have babies until they are in to their mid- to late-30s or even early 40s and beyond. Fortunately, these days, such events can usually be safely accommodated. But you must understand that, while laws exist to prevent age discrimination, nature can, and does, discriminate. After the age of 35, women are at an increased risk of having babies with chromosomal abnormalities such as Down syndrome. The miscarriage rate, again due to the age of the eggs, is also elevated significantly. Pregnancy complications such as high blood pressure, pregnancy-associated diabetes, and babies that are small for gestational age also increase substantially.

The older you get, the lower your chances for conceiving and the higher your risks for having a miscarriage or a baby with chromosomal abnormalities. You would be surprised at the number of highly educated women in their 40s and 50s who assume that, because they have regular periods, they can still have a baby. If you are in your 30s, these biological realities should be kept in mind. If the option to reproduce is not there for you, consider freezing your eggs or embryos with donor sperm (aka fertility preservation). If you are in your 40s, consider using donor eggs.

If you are lucky enough to conceive and make it through the first part of pregnancy with a "healthy" fetus, still remember that your body is older than that of the majority of women who have babies, even if you eat well and exercise regularly. You may be exceptionally healthy for a 40-year-old, but you are still a 40-year-old. However, you will likely have the benefit of being able to afford needed assistance. You will need extra testing. You will likely need to be delivered before your due date, especially if you are over 40. You will be at more risk for cesarean delivery because of complications and/or a 40-year-old uterus. You will be more at risk for having difficulties nursing. You will be more tired than the 20- to 30-year-old moms. Your parents will be older than their parents and thus not as likely to be able or willing to assist you in caring for your baby. This is not to discourage you from proceeding with your plans. Rather, it is to give you a heads up that many things change as you become "less young," and you are truly fortunate to be able to have a baby at this time in your life and should accept that honor and proceed with grace.

When Things Go Wrong

Sadly, not all pregnancies result in beautiful bouncing baby boys or girls. Many end in miscarriages, abnormal pregnancies like ectopic pregnancies, or with detected chromosomal or genetic abnormalities.

If you start to bleed or develop pain during the first trimester, contact your provider immediately. These signs are not necessarily harbingers of doom, but they may be associated with miscarriage or otherwise abnormal pregnancies. Sonograms and blood levels of the pregnancy hormone, human chorionic gonadotrophin (HCG), can help determine if the pregnancy is viable. If your pregnancy has developed to a certain point and then stops growing, or if it is located in your fallopian tube or other non-uterine position, you will not end up with the desired healthy baby.

If the pregnancy develops in your fallopian tubes or in another position outside of the uterus, it not only cannot survive, but you can develop life-threatening bleeding if you are left untreated. Medical and surgical options exist for this, and the choice will be determined by your particular situation.

If studies determine that your pregnancy is no longer viable, you will be given options that include letting nature take its course, medical therapies, or surgical interventions depending on how far along the pregnancy is. Generally, none of these options will have any impact on your future ability to conceive or carry a pregnancy to term. Nature, however, can be very wasteful when it comes to pregnancy. So many things can go wrong in the first few weeks. Step number 2,352 in a list of thousands may occur before step 2,340 or something called "nondisjunction" can occur in the division of an egg and result in an abnormal pregnancy that cannot survive. Up to 20 percent of recognized pregnancies end in miscarriage, more if you count chemical and unrecognized pregnancies, which are positive pregnancy tests without the development of a recognizable fetus.

Nothing short of drugs or surgical intervention can cause an otherwise healthy woman with a healthy pregnancy to miscarry. Staying up late at night, lifting something heavy, being stressed, having sex, thinking bad thoughts about your mother — none of these things cause you to miscarry. The older you are when you conceive, the higher the risk of loss. The good news is, you are not to blame for this loss. The bad news is, there is nothing you can do to prevent this from happening again.

Family and friends may try to comfort you by advising that you can always have another one (pregnancy). While that may or may not be true, especially if you are older or required IVF, you can no longer have THIS one. The moment you know you are pregnant; your mind skips forward to school plays and high school graduations and grandchildren. That's just what happens. The loss of potential is a full and real loss, not one to be discounted.

In the years I have practiced, I have come to notice a pattern. Mind you, not everyone fits into the generalization I am about to describe, but I have found that, in general, during the process of managing the medical issues associated with miscarriage, couples tend to do well together. They hold each other up and grieve together.

Unfortunately, after the loss, I have noted that women need to talk about it—a lot. It helps them heal. Men, on the other hand, tend not to want to talk about it. They feel bad about not being able to protect their partner or their unborn child and want, more than anything else, to not talk about it. Both forms of grieving make sense to the unbiased observer.

The problem occurs when couples hold each other at fault for the way they grieve. The woman may feel resentful and unappreciated if her partner will not talk with her about the loss. The man may be aggravated by what he sees as incessant talking about something unspeakable. The result is that, at a time when they both need the other for support, they are distanced from each other, each suffering not only the loss of their future, but also the loss of their partner.

There is no good or bad way to grieve. We grieve as we grieve. Knowing this, women might opt to talk more with their girlfriends or family members and men might allow a bit more discussion than they otherwise might have wanted to allow both to heal.

There will be several weeks of profound sadness, as is expected. Support groups are plentiful. Eventually, both should be able to move on. Allow one or two normal cycles to proceed, and then you may try again if you wish.

If a genetic, chromosomal, or structural anomaly is discovered, there follows, for some, the agonizing decision of whether or not to terminate the pregnancy. I will not go into the pros and cons of that choice. There is much to be said elsewhere about this, and this book is not the forum for such a discussion. Medically speaking, however, should a woman choose to terminate her pregnancy, there are options that are safe and that should have no effect on her future ability to conceive and carry a child to term.

Practicalities

Childcare

This may seem like an odd subject to be addressed in the first trimester section, but, if you are considering daycare, many childcare centers require you to sign up as soon as you have a due date in order to be considered for a position six months to a year after your baby is born. If you do not have a sibling in the daycare center, a generous maternity leave option at work, or family members in the area to step in for you when you return to work, this is the time to start interviewing and signing up. You may have to sign up for a few in order to increase your odds. Make sure to call when you have your baby to update the centers and reconfirm your interest.

Second Trimester

Congratulations! You have made it through the testiest part of your pregnancy. Your baby now has all of the rudiments of its major organ systems and is going about growing and maturing. If you have not already done so, you will soon be able to share your secret, and likely your baby's gender, with friends and family.

Medical Stuff

Weight Gain

Your visits to the doctor will include weight checks, which may be humbling indeed. Truly excessive weight gain, especially on top of pre-pregnancy Body Mass Index (BMI) over 30, which is considered obese, can be harmful to the pregnancy. For most women, though, excessive weight gain is more a matter of discomfort and concern about what will happen after the pregnancy.

The rules of calories in and calories out are not suspended during pregnancy. If you eat more than you did before you were pregnant and exercise less, you will gain weight. If you eat more than the recommended 350–450 calories and/or exercise less, you will gain more than is required for the baby, amniotic fluid, placenta, and breast tissue. Nature does not provide a dispensation for pregnancy in terms of weight gain. Like it or not, the amount that you gain (except for those with excessive fluid retention, which is, in fact, a small minority) is based on the number of calories in and the number of calories burned. While you will likely not cause harm to your pregnancy or yourself if you overshoot, that weight will remain on your hips and thighs after you deliver. The choice is yours.

Genetic Testing

The 16-week visit is the time for many to get a final test for structural or chromosomal anomalies. The AFP, AFP Plus, or the Tetrascreen tests use maternal blood, the results of a special ultrasound, and maternal age and race to calculate the odds that a particular baby has a chromosomal abnormality. If the risk is higher than that of a 35-year-old, further testing with cell-free fetal DNA will be recommended. If that test is abnormal as well, amniocentesis will be offered. The tests can also determine if your baby is at higher risk for having a neural tube defect (structural abnormality of the spinal cord or brain) or complications later in the pregnancy, such as pregnancy-associated blood pressure elevation, preeclampsia (blood pressure elevation with or without protein in the urine), or fetal growth restriction (small for dates babies). All of these complications result in an increased risk of the need to deliver the mother earlier to avoid the potential for stillbirth or significant maternal complications.

At 20 weeks, a special ultrasound, known as the anatomy scan, is performed to look for structural abnormalities. During this scan, you should be able to see the four chambers of the heart, the kidneys, the limbs, the hands (often with the thumb being sucked), and major features of the brain, even if you don't know what they are.

Gestational Diabetes

At 24 weeks, testing is done for gestational diabetes, or pregnancy associated blood sugar elevations. First, you will be given a sugary drink to
consume. Then your blood will be drawn an hour later. If the glucose level
is elevated, meaning you failed this "screen," you will be asked to take a
formal test for diabetes known as the glucose tolerance test, or GTT. If this
too is abnormal, a dietitian will counsel you, place you on a special meal
plan, and teach you how to monitor your blood sugars at home.

Women with gestational diabetes who do not receive appropriate treatment
during their pregnancies are at an increased risk of having large babies at
term, which can result in labor complications or necessitate the need for a
cesarean delivery. Your baby may also need to be monitored after birth and
potentially given an IV with glucose in it to stabilize his or her blood sugar.

Women who develop gestational diabetes are at increased risk of developing it in subsequent pregnancies and have an elevated overall lifetime risk
of developing type 2 diabetes.

The biggest milestone of the second trimester is at 24 weeks. At this point,
your baby can survive if born. This is not to say that there may not be medical concerns if that happens, but you will likely have a take-home prize if
you deliver at or beyond 24 weeks.

When Things Go Wrong

The second trimester is generally a relatively eventless, if not prolonged,
time in pregnancy. However, there are some known problems that can
occur.

If you have had three or more elective pregnancy terminations or dilation
and curettages (D&C), a second trimester termination, or either a Loop
Electrical Excision Procedure (LEEP), or cone biopsy to remove precancerous cells from your cervix, you may be at risk for developing something
called an incompetent cervix. With an incompetent cervix, the cervix pain-

lessly dilates after 16 weeks of pregnancy. The result is that you may end up delivering your baby before it can survive outside the womb. Women with this history are monitored carefully with regular sonograms that evaluate the length of the cervix. Should premature shortening or dilation occur, you may be put on bed rest, have a pessary (a flexible device that is placed in the vagina for support) placed, or have a stitch, called a cerclage, placed in the cervix to help keep the baby inside until a safer time.

In the event that a chromosomal abnormality is detected after your Ultra-Screen test or a lethal, or potentially lethal, anomaly is noted during the anatomy screen, a decision will have to be made as to whether or not to continue the pregnancy.

Preterm delivery can also occur, although the cause is frequently not known. The rate in the United States increased to 9.8 percent in 2016. The most common cause is previous preterm labor (1.5 to 2-fold increase risk in subsequent pregnancy), which, in itself is not very helpful information. Medications exist that attempt to stop contractions and potent steroids can be given, if necessary, to help mature the baby's lungs in the event that delivery cannot be delayed. Fortunately, these events are not that frequent.[29]

Practicalities

Many women, especially those over 35, choose to wait until their Ultra-Screen test at 16 weeks or their 20-week anatomy scan before sharing with others that they are pregnant. If this is your first pregnancy, that might not be too difficult to do, however, if your body has previously been torn asunder by a baby, you might not be able to hide it this long.

Maternity Clothing

This is the time when you may find that you no longer fit your regular clothes but are still too small to justify wearing maternity clothes. I liken it to adolescence when your body is no longer that of a child but still quite

---

29. Committee Opinion, 2012.

a way from that of a woman. You can choose to "suck it in" and be uncomfortable if you wish. I find that this happens more in first pregnancies. Regardless, at some point, you will realize that comfort is more important than image.

There are many options for oversized and early pregnancy clothes. If you are lucky, you will have friends who have clothes to lend you. Recycling is the way to go, not only for the environment, but for your budget as well. If you insist on hiding as long as you can, know that you cannot harm your baby by wearing clothes that are too tight. You will be miserable, but cute, and your baby will be fine. It's sort of like wearing high heels to walk to work when you could wear sneakers or flip-flops.

When making your list of "must-haves" for your wardrobe, please consider including the following:

1) A belly band to extend the life (and waist) of your pre-pregnancy pants and skirts when you are no longer able to zip them up but would look ridiculous in maternity clothes.

2) Maternity jeans. These are a must, but well-fitting ones, like regular jeans, are difficult to find. Order a few different kinds and be prepared to return some.

3) Leggings. The more, the merrier. They are so comfortable and so forgiving.

4) Long tank tops. A dangling underbelly is never sexy. Flowing tops for early pregnancy work when you look more fat than pregnant.

5) Machine-washable tops. Your ever-enlarging belly becomes a magnet for food, especially in the latter part of pregnancy.

6) Cute flats. Heels, while cute, became a hazard as you get into the third trimester.

7) Wrap dresses are always nice. Look for those, as well as black fitted dresses that you can accessorize in various ways to extend your wardrobe.

8) A nice pair of maternity pajamas. Sleeping is already disrupted enough with pregnancy. You don't need uncomfortable sleepwear as well.

9) If you are going to pump, consider getting a bra that allows for both breastfeeding and pumping when you are in your third trimester and your breasts have reached their maximum pregnancy size. This will save you from buying bras for the last part of pregnancy that will not be useful after delivery.

10) You will likely be nursing much longer than you will need to wear maternity clothes, so look into combo tops to accommodate this.

Nursery

Once the reality of your pregnancy and all that it entails settles in, a sort of panic tends to occur. You realize that you need to get things ready for your little one. The number of "must-haves" is truly mind-boggling. You could spend a literal fortune on nursery items and clothing. If you have a lot of discretionary income, go for it. If not, Target and Bed, Bath and Beyond will soon become your new best friends.

Hopefully, you will have at least one friend who has made this journey before and will clue you in as to what is truly necessary. Or, if you are an over-achieving millennial, you will have at least one friend with a spreadsheet containing all manner of car seats, cribs, strollers, etc. to compare.

If you want to keep it simple, I encourage parents-to-be to pretend that they live in a one- or two-bedroom apartment in Manhattan and have minimal room to expand. Women who live there have babies every day and do just fine.

While this is a generality, I have noticed that men tend to focus more on long-term concerns, such as college tuition which, given the realities of education costs today, is a huge issue, while women tend to focus more on the practicalities of the short-term, like decorating the nursery. Please don't take offense if your spouse is not so interested in the color scheme of the nursery or matching crib sheets and wall decorations; he is just as excited about the baby as you are, just not so much concerned about the room in which the infant will sleep.

Childcare

The second trimester is the time to solidify plans for childcare. Sadly, many daycare centers require you to sign up as soon as you have a due date. If you don't plan to put your baby in daycare, please start to consider nannies, nanny shares, au pairs, or family members. Do the legwork now. It will save you plenty of time and worry when you are home on maternity leave. This is also the time to solidify with your place of work just how much time you will have off. Absolutely do not agree to start working from home after a brief period of time because, after all, the baby sleeps most of the time, right? Wrong! You will be sleep deprived and need to clean, cook, shower— all the things a normal functioning human needs to accomplish.

Belly Bumps and Unsolicited Advice

Whenever you begin to show, be prepared for people who feel the need to touch your belly or offer advice about what you should or shouldn't be doing during your pregnancy. Do not be afraid to tell them you don't wish to be touched if you find it inappropriate. Have some witty retorts ready, if you wish, for those people in Starbucks who advise you that coffee is not good for your baby. As mentioned in a previous section, if you wish to imbibe, please consider doing so in private, as the world tends to feel entitled to "protect" your baby. If someone says something to you about you smoking, well, you deserve that.

Childbirth Preparation Classes

While it may seem too early to sign up for classes, you might want to consider starting your research now, especially if you want a natural childbirth. Many classes fill up early. More about this later in the Third Trimester section.

Breast Pumps

The Affordable Care Act provides the availability of electric breast pumps for all new mothers in order to promote breastfeeding. Generally, you can order a breast pump after 28 weeks of pregnancy (in which case, you can check this off your list early), although some insurance companies request that you wait until your baby is born and then have it delivered to your house. Please look into the specific requirements of your plan.

The options for breast pumps are staggering. Will you simply need your pump at home, or will you need it at work, or when you are commuting? Believe it or not, there are pumps and bras for all of these options. Most insurance companies cover Medela pumps, however, the Spectra pump seems to be gaining popularity. Also, Willow is a new hands-free bra option that has gotten a lot of good press lately. Large organizations like Kaiser may supply you with their own preferred brand that may or may not be sufficient for anything other than the occasional emptying of your breasts before you go out. Sadly, there are no silent pumps yet, so if you will be working from home, consider not pumping when talking to a perspective client or trying to seal a deal. They can hear you! Even if they don't realize what you're doing.

Third Trimester

This is it! At some point very soon, you are going to officially be somebody's mother. From 28 weeks on, you are considered to be in your third trimester. Everything is formed, it's just not mature. Your baby's brain grows the most during this last trimester, and his or her lungs become developed enough to live outside the womb. If you make it to 37 weeks, all should be well with your baby, although there may be a few hiccups along the way. By 39 weeks, you should definitely have a take-home prize.

Medical Concerns

The third trimester is fraught with risks like stillbirth, pregnancy-related high blood pressure, preeclampsia or eclampsia (disorders associated with blood pressure elevation, protein in the urine, and, potentially, seizures when severe), fetal growth restriction, or small-for-dates babies that are at risk for stillbirth, cholestasis of pregnancy (a gallbladder disorder specific to pregnancy), etc. For details on these issues, you should peruse books intended to inform (okay, terrify) you about all of these possibilities, but please, *please* be careful about those sites on the internet intended to frighten you about all things related to pregnancy.

For the purposes of this book, suffice it to say that while most women do well, there are a number of things that can and do go wrong in pregnancy in the third trimester. That's the bad news. The good news is that, if necessary, your baby can usually be delivered early to prevent dire consequences. Hence the reason for more frequent visits at the end of pregnancy.

From 28 to 35 or 36 weeks, you will be seen every two weeks. After that point, until the end of pregnancy, you will be seen on a weekly basis. Your blood pressure, urine, and weight will be checked regularly to look for signs of medical complications, and your baby's size will be assessed either with a tape measure or a sonogram, depending on your circumstances, to document adequate growth.

Fluid Retention

Sudden and significant weight gain or blood pressure elevation can signal the development of hypertensive disorders such as preeclampsia or pregnancy-induced hypertension. These can affect the growth of your baby and put you at risk for serious complications necessitating early delivery. To confuse the picture, many women put on a lot of weight in the last trimester because they retain fluid. Fluid retention is natural to some degree in the last part of pregnancy, and some women have a predisposition for this. However, ingesting too much salt can aggravate this tendency. Other women start to retain fluid because they are overweight to begin with or gain too much weight during pregnancy. Take an honest assessment of your diet. If the majority of what you eat is either boxed, bagged, canned, deli'd, frozen, or fast, you are likely consuming excessive amounts of salt, which can result in, at the very least, misery and discomfort, and, at worst, sustained blood pressure elevation.

If you have the misfortune of being pregnant in the summer in a southern state, you will certainly face swollen ankles and hands. You might even develop what has lovingly been referred to as "cankles," or uniform swelling of the legs from the knees down. To minimize this, avoid the above-mentioned foods and drink a lot of water. Elevate your feet above the level of your heart (not the same as putting them up on a stool!) a few times a day. As soon as you get home in the evenings, after emptying your bladder, find your couch, take off your shoes, and elevate your feet for 15 or 20 minutes before proceeding with your evening. Believe me, whatever is left undone during those few moments can wait. Your comfort is more important. Compression stockings that go to the top of your thighs will be helpful here as well.

If you suddenly put on five or more pounds, your face is swollen, you are feeling generally not well, or you develop a severe headache that does not respond to over-the-counter medications, call your doctor, as these can be signs of severe preeclampsia or pregnancy-induced hypertension that may require you to be delivered immediately.

Final Tests and Vaccinations

A final blood draw and cultures will be done at 36 weeks to determine whether your blood count is adequate for delivery or if you need more iron. You will be tested again for sexually transmitted diseases and treated if positive. You will also be tested for a bacterium that many women carry in their reproductive or urinary tract called beta strep. If you test positive, you will be given an antibiotic during labor to protect your baby from this bacterium. There is no point in giving it at the time of the diagnosis because you are colonized, not infected, and the bacteria cannot be eradicated from your system.

You will be advised to have a Tdap (tetanus, diphtheria, and pertussis) shot to protect your baby from pertussis. Your partner and grandparents and babysitters and anyone else that will be around your baby on a regular basis will be asked to get a shot as well if they haven't done so in the last 10 years.

Pertussis is a disease that had almost been eradicated in this country until, subsequently proven to be false, data was put out there to suggest that the vaccine could cause autism. This simply is not the case. What is the case is that babies are now dying needlessly of a disease that does not have to exist.

In the same vein, influenza can be devastating to pregnant women, sometimes landing them in the intensive care unit if infected. If you are or will be pregnant during flu season, please get vaccinated. And partners and family members, please get your vaccinations as well. You do not want to infect the baby.

Practical Considerations

Preparing for Labor

By 32 weeks, it will dawn on you that this little one will soon need to make an exit. You might look at your now not-so-tiny belly and begin to panic as you contemplate the very small size of your vagina. Childbirth classes are helpful at this point as you will learn that delivery is a very natural thing indeed. While painful, it is a doable process.

If you are one of those people who are absolutely certain that you want an epidural as soon as you arrive at the hospital, sign up for the short series of classes that go over the ins and outs of labor and delivery.

If you are planning to have a natural delivery, you might want to sign up for more extensive training. Understand though, that no matter how much education you obtain, there will be some pain associated with the process. If you attend a class and are told that the various methods about to be taught will make your childbirth painless, run, don't walk, to the nearest exit. Yes, there are breathing exercises and other tools to help you through the process, but nothing short of an epidural will take away the pain. If you think it will, you will be setting yourself up for disappointment.

Epidural

I distinctly remember a very angry husband a few years ago, who made sure to let me know that he was a lawyer, literally yelling at me that his wife was experiencing 9 out of 10 pain according to the chart by her bed during her natural childbirth. The implication was that there was something I could, and should, do to prevent this. I advised that she could have an epidural, which they didn't want, or continue on their chosen path. He argued that it wasn't fair; no, it isn't, but that is the way it is. We did not design this process but do our best to make it safe and tolerable for the mother and baby.

Options to control pain in labor were developed for a reason. It hurts—a lot! Sadly, the initial choices were a medication called scopolamine, which was used in doses so large that it robbed women of their sense of reality and took away their ability to participate in the process, or the older epidurals, which were really quite awful. Huge doses of anesthetic were given every three to four hours, resulting in profound numbness, nausea, vomiting, and, often, decreases in the baby's heart rate that required oxygen administration and maternal repositioning, not to mention anxiety over what was happening to the baby. This was followed by a sudden and complete absence of effect after a few hours and 20–30 minutes of significant discomfort before becoming profoundly numb again. And so, the cycle would repeat. Once a woman was completely dilated, no more medication could be given, and women had to push while adjusting to the pain. All of this made women think twice about trying to intervene in this process, and thus, the development of natural childbirth classes. Fortunately, current epidurals are continuous and far less profound in terms of their effect. The dose can even be adjusted based on the stage of labor a woman is in when she receives it, allowing her to push effectively with good pain relief until the very end when not much in this universe can protect you from that final exit. But then it is over, and you have your baby in your arms. You won't even notice that your doctor is repairing any "alterations" to your bottom that may have resulted from the dramatic exit. If you end up opting for an epidural, you should not be made to feel you have failed.

There is some nebulous information out there that epidurals can cause paralysis. Suffice it to say that, after 40 years of practice, I don't know anybody who knows anybody who knows anybody who has had this happen.

At this point, I cannot help but share two stories. The first is about the first labor I participated in as a medical student. The mother was British and had had two babies already. Unfortunately, her husband was out of country at the time of her labor, and she was alone. When I came into the room, she was reading a book. Every three minutes or so, she put the book down on her belly, closed her eyes, and breathed softly. She would then pick the book up and start reading again. After a while, I asked her if she was experiencing any pain. Her calm reply was, "It's excruciating, really." Shortly after, she delivered a healthy seven-pound baby with no anesthesia. I was amazed.

The other story is of a very sweet couple in early labor. They had plans for a natural childbirth, but as the wife got into the active phase of labor, around 4 centimeters dilated, she began to get uncomfortable. She mentioned something about an epidural to her husband, who reminded her that "we" had agreed she would do this without medication. I left them alone to discuss this. At this point, there arrived on Labor and Delivery, what we in the field call a "stop and drop," a woman who had delivered before and was completely dilated upon arrival. Needless to say, there was a lot of noise for about 10 to 15 minutes and then silence, followed by the cry of a healthy baby. Shortly after the delivery, I went into the room to check on the couple. The husband was curled up in the fetal position on a couch by the window looking terrified.

"What in the hell was that?" he asked.

"That, sir, was natural childbirth," I replied.

"It sounded like a pterodactyl! Please don't let that happen to my wife!" he pleaded.

She received an epidural and delivered, quietly and happily, some six hours later.

Many of my patients have been pleasantly surprised at how well they did without medication, either by choice or by accident. Others have vowed they would never again do it without pain medication. This is YOUR labor, and, barring any significant medical complications, it should be yours to experience in the way you wish.

Perineal Massage

If you are told to perform perineal massage to prepare your vagina for labor, you might want to consider watching a movie with your spouse or going for an evening stroll instead. The likelihood that you could put enough pressure on your bottom to prepare for childbirth is minuscule. If you are willing to roll a bowling ball through the area, you might come close to preparing. If you have ever seen a delivery, you will know that the space between your vagina and rectum becomes literally paper thin prior to delivery of the head. I can't imagine normal and emotionally-stable people stretching their private parts to such a limit prior to delivery.

Nipple Preparation

The idea that you can prepare your nipples for breastfeeding prior to delivery is a bit of a fantasy as well. One of my fellow residents who had had a baby once suggested that the only way to really prepare would be to take a vacuum cleaner hose and attach it to your nipples. Not going to happen.

To Shave or Not To Shave

Should you shave prior to delivery? Only if you generally shave or wax. Otherwise, leave nature to nature. Your doctor really does not care how you look, and the baby will come out one way or the other.

Doula

Do you want a doula? For some, this is a very practical, if not expensive, option. Make sure you find someone who will work with you and your needs and is not there to defy the medical world and "protect" you from their interventions. It would help if she had some medical training as well, not just the experience of having delivered a baby or two herself. Also, remember that the doula should assist you and your partner. She is not, and should not, be there to take the place of your significant other, unless, of course, yours is deployed or otherwise unavailable.

Birthing Plans

Many childbirth preparation classes and websites offer prefabricated, fill-in-the-blank birthing plans. If you feel the need to draw one up, have at it and discuss it with your provider. Please know, however, that they have likely seen various permutations of your plan and are not really learning anything from your suggestions. If you have neither the time nor the inclination to draw up such a form, don't worry about it. It's not required. However, if there are issues that are very important to you, please take the time to discuss these in detail with your provider during the latter part of your pregnancy.

Home Delivery

This book is not the forum to go into the pros and cons of birth away from a medical facility that offers support to the mother and newborn when the unexpected occurs. Suffice it to say though, that delivery is a messy business. There is the amniotic fluid, a unit or two of your blood, urine, and stool to contend with. There is also the vomit that occurs as you enter the active phase of labor and begin pushing. In my humble opinion, these are things you don't want to do in your own home. Nor do you want to expose your fancy pillows and cases and your pricey pajamas to this effluvium. When delivering in a traditional environment, wear and use what the hospital provides. You can get cute after delivery if you want to entertain your guests. While I never minded the "presents" I received during deliveries, as those come with the territory, I personally wore what the nurses referred to as a hazmat suit—a full-sized plastic suit and a mask with a visor—for all of my deliveries after years of having amniotic fluid and blood on my legs, vomit on my face, and other such delicacies applied to various other parts of my body.

Cord Blood Banking

If you have ordered even one thing online related to your pregnancy or impending baby, you will start receiving information about cord blood banking to store potentially life-saving fetal stem cells for future need. After delivery and delayed cord clamping, fetal blood can be drawn from the umbilical cord, processed, frozen, and stored indefinitely.

While there are a few genetic disorders that have improved from the use of fetal stem cells, blood from the affected baby cannot be used to treat that baby's disorder, although it could potentially be used for a sibling. Much research is being done on the use of fetal stem cell for conditions like cerebral palsy and Alzheimer's disease, and promising "effects" have been seen in a number of studies. However, one should not count on this as an insurance policy.

Currently, the collection, processing, and freezing of cord blood costs about $2,000, with an additional annual fee of a few hundred dollars for storage. This is not covered by any insurance plan. When you add this to the non-insurance costs for maternity care, maternity wardrobe, nursery items, diapers, etc. this option, for most, becomes a luxury. When my patients ask me about storing cord blood, my advice is the following: if you have a lot of discretionary income and/or you are an anxious person, do it. If not, buy a car seat with the money. That makes more sense. You could also choose to donate the blood to a public bank. There is no need to waste precious biological material that has the potential to positively affect another child's life. You will not be charged for this, but you also will not have access to that blood should the unlikely need arise in the future.

Currently, the American College of Obstetricians and Gynecologists encourages providers to discuss cord blood banking in a balanced way if information is requested. Some states now even mandate this. However, it discourages providers from routinely offering this option as a "biological insurance policy."[30]

Labor. This Is It!

One of the most annoying calls I received as an obstetrician was from my patients' husbands announcing that "we" are in labor. Make no mistake about it. YOU, as the husband, are not in labor. Your wife is. As such, it is best, unless she is incapacitated or unable to speak English, that she talks to the physician when the call needs to be made. Only she can answer all of the necessary questions.

There are a number of complicated algorithms you can use to determine if you're in labor. I have found that the best rule of thumb is, if your contractions have been predictably 3 to 5 minutes apart for an hour, it is probable that whatever is happening is likely to end in the delivery of your baby. This is a good time to call and speak with your physician. If you are comfortable enough to remain at home, if the membranes have not ruptured (water has not broken), and the baby is moving, there is room to negotiate. For example, if it is rush hour or you live fairly close to the hospital, you might want to stay at home for a while. The average length of the first labor, like it or not, is 12 to 20 hours. If your beta strep culture was positive at 36 weeks and/or you note meconium-stained amniotic fluid (evidence of the fetus having had a bowel movement in utero), you will be advised to go to the hospital right away.

Upon arrival, you and your baby will be monitored. Your cervix will be checked to see if there is a change from when you were last seen in the office. If it is determined that you are in labor, you will be admitted for further monitoring.

---

30. Committee Opinion, 2015.

In general, labor is the time for you and you partner to work together to bring your baby into the world. If family members and friends want to be present, be cognizant of the fact that this is not a spectator sport. If they are there to support you and your partner, that's great, but if you feel the need to entertain them, have your nurse be the bad guy and ask them to leave. Grandmothers, unless asked, this is not the time to talk about your labor experiences. Really. Nobody wants to hear about that. And please don't remind your daughter, or especially your daughter-in-law, who gets an epidural after hours of labor, that you popped your babies out with nothing but love.

The early part of labor, or the latent phase, covers the first 4 to 6 cm of cervical dilation. This phase of labor can take a long time, up to 12 or more hours in some cases (or longer if you are being induced). How long it lasts is not a determining factor of the total length of your labor. Toward the end of this first phase, you will begin to get very uncomfortable. You may get nauseated and throw up. You might lose your sense of humor, and your partner may no longer look cute to you or be amusing. That's a good sign though; it means that you are moving on to the active phase of labor.

From this point forward, dilation is more predictable. For first babies, you generally dilate 1+ cm an hour going forward. For second or more babies, the process is much faster.

This is generally the time when women must decide whether or not they want pain medication. If you are progressing quickly, you might benefit from instructed breathing or other methods to help you tolerate the painful process. If your labor isn't moving quickly or you know that you want pain medication, this is the perfect time to request an epidural; it is not as likely to slow the progress of your labor at this time.

If you suddenly feel that you can't take the pain any more or you start vomiting and feeling an urge to bear down, this is good news, as it likely means that you are almost completely dilated and ready to enter the second stage of labor. At this point, you will need to push with contractions to help your baby exit the birth canal. Sadly, many childbirth classes tend to fast forward this part of the process with the implication that it is fairly quick. For baby number two or more, it is indeed usually a short period of time, about 5 to 20 minutes. For first babies though, this process can, and usually does, take one to two or more hours of very hard work to bring the baby through and out of the vagina.

Once your baby is delivered, barring complications, he or she will be placed on your abdomen. Current recommendations are to let the cord stop pulsating before clamping it.[31] If everything is going well, your partner will be allowed to cut the cord. You should then have time to hold and get to know your baby while bothersome, but necessary, medical issues are tended to, like assessing the baby's vital signs and determining Apgar Scores, a measure of how the baby is doing and whether or not resuscitative measures are needed.

Other necessities include the delivery of your placenta and repair of any tears or cuts to your perineum. In the way distant past, episiotomies, or cuts to the perineum, were performed automatically to "ease" the delivery of your baby. This is no longer the case. Study after study has proven that "preventive" cuts are not only unnecessary but can lead to an increased amount of extended tearing of your perineum that results in significant discomfort postpartum. That being said, given the size of most babies born today, the likelihood that your bottom will be completely intact after delivery of your first seven pound infant (or larger) is small. Tears can, and likely will, happen unless your baby is small, about five to six pounds. The good news is that, while they may be more difficult for your obstetrician to repair, most of these spontaneous tears are more "user-friendly" to your body, meaning they are more likely to involve the vaginal rather than the perineal tissue and thus cause you less discomfort in the postpartum period. You will be given a local anesthetic to numb the area for necessary repairs if you did not have an epidural.

---

31. Committee Opinion, 2017.

When Things Go Wrong

The goal of most women is to have an eventless, swift and relatively pain-free vaginal delivery of a healthy, take-home baby. Trying to go into the realities of things like premature delivery, still birth, compromised babies, or severe maternal complications necessitating extended and complex medical care in this book would do an injustice to those who have these things occur. For that, I refer you to those books that are written to address these issues or, even better, to your obstetrician or maternal fetal medicine specialist.

What I will address is the very real possibility that your labor may take longer than planned, especially if you need to be induced for medical reasons, hurt more than you expected, or that, at some point it will be determined that you need to deliver by cesarean section or have an assisted vaginal delivery by vacuum or forceps.

Many women are suspicious of the medical world and believe there is much too much intervention into an otherwise natural process. It is true that the United States has an unacceptably high cesarean section rate, especially when you compare our infant mortality rate with those of other countries. Believe it or not, much research and teaching of residents and practicing physicians is being done by the American College of Obstetricians and Gynecologists to lower this number significantly.

That being said, there are occasions when the use of Pitocin (a drug used to induce or augment labor), assisted vaginal delivery (using vacuum or forceps), or cesarean delivery may become necessary for your health or that of your baby. It is important to feel comfortable discussing these issues with your physician. Hopefully, you have found someone who will listen to your needs and concerns. That way, if these things occur, you can have confidence that the right decisions are being made and your preferences are being considered. But remember, your idea of the ideal labor and delivery is actually not the goal of this entire process. The goal is the safe delivery of a healthy baby to a healthy mother. Whether you delivered naturally, with drugs, or by cesarean matters little when you are pushing your baby in a swing next to a mother who may have delivered in a different way.

Many couples have the preformed notion that Pitocin, which is a synthetic version of what your body makes in labor to affect delivery, will harm your baby or make your labor worse than it otherwise would be and thus should be avoided at all costs. I've seen the website that shows a hapless baby in a uterus being squeezed to death by Pitocin. Truth be told, that same cartoon could be used in a video of what happens in natural childbirth, as it's difficult to get a baby out of a uterus. But that is good news, because we don't want them dropping in the street willy-nilly at any point in the pregnancy! Pitocin also does not cause autism or any other harm to the baby. In fact, refusing the use of Pitocin when your doctor recommends it may result in your baby developing an infection or an unnecessary cesarean delivery.

Pitocin is generally recommended when your body's natural efforts are not sufficient to affect delivery, i.e. you are not in adequate labor. Pitocin puts you in adequate labor, which hurts a lot. The goal is to have your labor pattern mimic that of someone in adequate spontaneous labor. Nature has figured out the safest and most effective way to do that, and that is what is aimed for when this medication is given. The total amount of force, the length of the contractions, and the peak pressure in millimeters of mercury are the same if naturally supplied, or supplied by manmade Pitocin. That being said, many people who have experienced labor both with Pitocin and without it often recount that the naturally occurring contractions seem to ease up to the peak and then ease down while Pitocin-induced contractions seem to go immediately to the peak and stay there the entire time.

Pitocin can be dangerous when used inappropriately. I liken it to fire. It can be used to warm and light your house, but, if left unattended, can burn it down. The same is true with Pitocin. It needs to be given judiciously and with constant monitoring. This means you will need to be attached (not "strapped," a word many childbirth instructors like to use) to a monitor. You will be able to move around for comfort, but you will not be able to walk the halls, something those in advanced labor rarely do.

Unfortunately, there are occasions when babies do not tolerate labor, and a decision will need to be made to expedite matters, either by an assisted vaginal delivery with forceps or a vacuum or by cesarean delivery. Again, your goal here should be a healthy baby and a healthy you. Discuss the indications and alternatives with your doctor and decide based on your particular situation and the risk or benefit to you or your baby rather than a preformed notion that these things are simply bad. You have not failed if you don't have the textbook labor and delivery. Yours and your baby's safety is far more important than that.

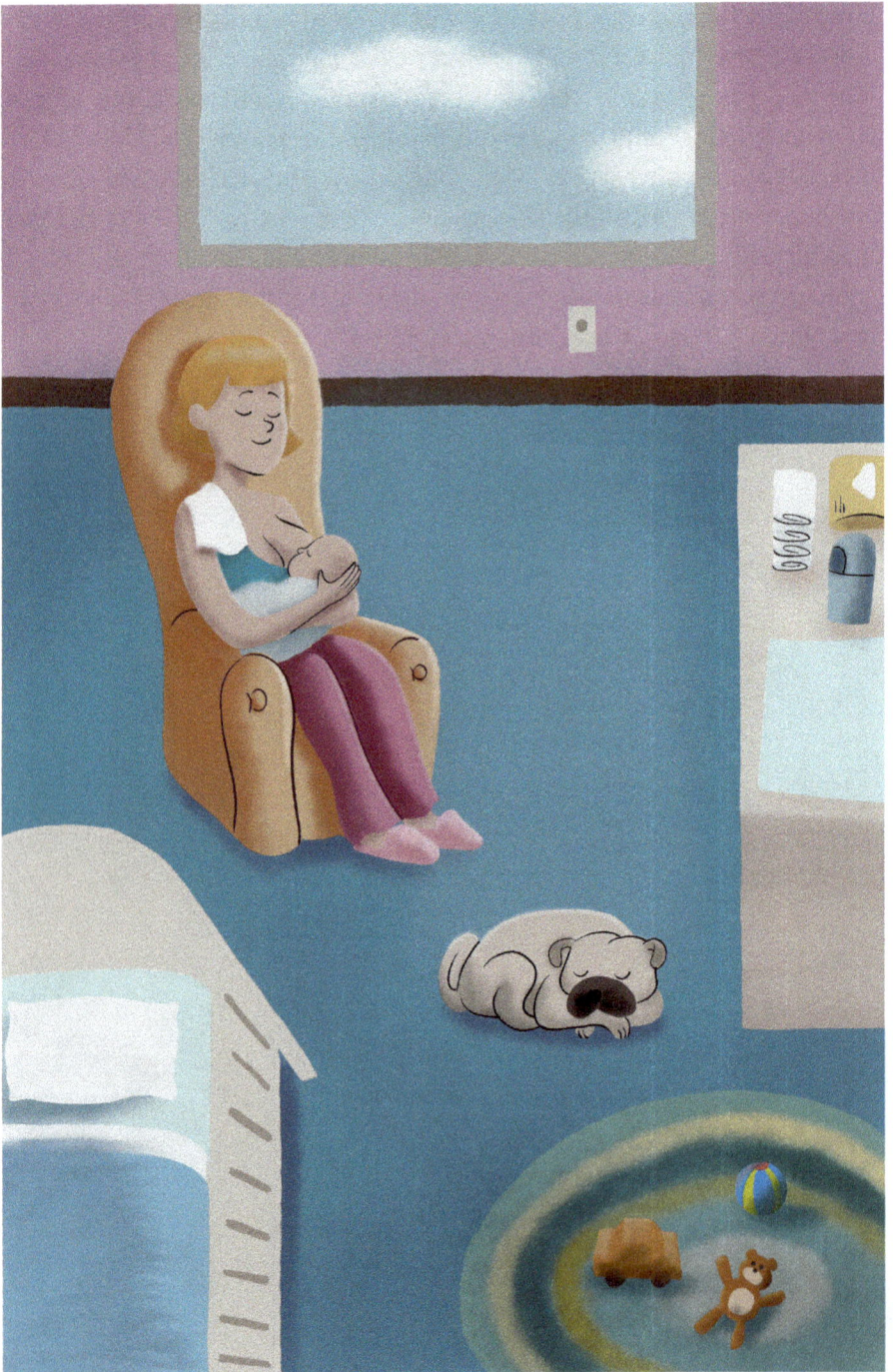

Part Three

Postpartum Considerations

Postpartum Stay

First and foremost, please remember that the time you spend in the hospital after you have your baby is for you to recover. You should not feel compelled to entertain guests, no matter how excited they may be to see you and your baby.

You have gone through nine months of discomfort and hours of pain. You are exhausted and have a sore bottom — or abdomen if you had a cesarean delivery. Visitors should be limited to immediate family and as few friends and associates as possible. These individuals should keep visits short and sweet. You need this time to recover and catch up as much as possible on your sleep. Try to remember, especially you first-time mothers, that the hospital personnel have a great deal of experience with babies. Believe it or not, there are one or two individuals on this earth that know what to do with and for your baby besides you.

A warning here, because this is something, I admit, I did not know about before my granddaughter was recently born. Many hospitals tout themselves as "baby friendly," meaning they encourage mother-baby bonding at all times. What that translated into for my daughter was her and her husband being left alone with their infant in the wee hours of the morning after two days of induction and labor with no meaningful sleep. They were beyond exhausted and had no option to put their baby in the nursery for a few hours to get some much-needed rest; there weren't any nurses there to tend to the baby! While I agree with the philosophy in principal, forcing sleepless individuals with no experience with babies to fend for themselves after the physical trauma of labor and hours, if not days, without sleep is not what I call "baby friendly." I whole-heartedly support mother-baby bonding when the mother is awake and aware enough to participate. Educated, rested, and supported moms and their babies benefit from uninterrupted time together.

Sibling Time

For you second- or third-time dads, I know you are tired when you get to the hospital because you have been taking care of the other children at home, but your visit to the hospital should not be the time for you to watch the game, read the paper, or get something to eat in the hospital cafeteria while you allow Mom to spend "quality time" with the older kids.

If this isn't your first child, you may feel some guilt because you are, in essence, cheating on your first or second with this newer and more exciting one. That's natural. The one you are holding is all potential. The one that comes to visit you is rife with memories and good times. Try to remember to take time with them alone after you get home. Anybody can hold or watch an infant sleep. Only you can spend that special quality time with your first or second. You will feel better, as will they.

Consider leaving the baby in the nursery when your first-born comes to visit. Spend time with him or her first. They have missed you. Then have your partner bring them to the nursery to see the baby and bring him or her to you. Maybe even have a gift for your first-born from the baby or from you when they arrive.

Push Gift

Some hapless partners are unaware that such a thing exists. The rest have fortunately been clued in either by their spouse or knowledgeable friends.

Personally, I think the term cheapens the intent. You are not being re-warded for pushing a baby out, certainly not if you had a cesarean section. Rather, the gift is the opportunity for your significant other to say thank you for carrying his or her child for nine months, for suffering through morning sickness, for being extraordinarily tired, for having your body morph into something unrecognizable, for getting stretch marks, and then, at the end, for subjecting yourself to labor and vaginal or surgical delivery, and then nursing your child. The gift is to say that they would have done it themselves, if possible, and that they are so very thankful you have done so for the two of you. As such, they would like to show you in a palpable way how much they appreciate you.

For partners, please understand that this gift should, in most cases, not be a practical one. It should not be something for the baby or for the nursery. It should be something extra for her to say thank you. In most cases, this translates into jewelry, although other treasures can be acceptable.

Ideally, the gift should be given while the mother is in the hospital, as something you thought about and planned for in advance. If you do not do so, she may not say anything at first. If you get home and still have not gotten the gift, there will eventually come an explosive time when your failure to have done so will become a huge issue. At that point, you can go out and buy something, but believe me; it can never be big enough or expensive enough to make up for the fact that you did not provide it when you should have. Don't like this? Too bad. YOU did not go through preg-nancy and delivery. SHE did.

Going Home

Once you are home, true friends will call with just enough time to allow you to brush your teeth and put something on that does not reek of spit up but not so much time that you feel compelled to clean your house. They should bring food and/or a gift, "ooh" and "ahh" at your baby, and then disappear after 30 minutes at the most. Also, you may wish to clue your unaware (or child-free) friends into some key points, such as not coming when they are sick, washing their hands before touching the baby, etc.

However, please do not provide a 30-point checklist for visitation rights unless your goal is to keep everyone away.

If you are truly lucky, you will either have helpful (not needy, pushy, or judgmental) family to actually assist when you get home or be that small percent of privileged individuals who are able to afford a night nurse. The first couple of weeks can be quite challenging, to say the least. Let's discuss a hypothetical situation here because it happens, a lot! You are exhausted. If this is your first baby, you are likely terrified and without a clue as to which of the bits of advice or online information to believe. This tiny person, who has stolen your heart in a way that you could never have imagined, needs you to hold and feed him or her on an unimaginable timescale. After a day or two, you cannot imagine going any further, and yet you must. Others have done it. Why can't you?

You've waited at least nine months for this, not including the time you spent trying to get pregnant. For those with infertility issues, a lot more time has been invested and postpartum sadness is far more likely. You expected to feel fulfilled and elated. Instead, you are exhausted. You are hormonal. Your body doesn't feel right. Your vagina hurts. You pee on yourself without warning. You are wearing pads, which many young women have never done before, and ridiculous hospital underwear. You are exhausted. Your baby keeps crying. Your partner seems useless. You cry because he is wearing something green or gray or blue. It doesn't matter. Your breast milk doesn't come in the way you expected. Your nipples are bleeding. Your guests irritate you. You wonder why you did this in the first place, but you are afraid to say anything because that would suggest that you are not appreciative of this wonderful blessing. You snap at you partner. You yell at your nurse. You are angry. You cry just because.

What's wrong with you? In most cases, absolutely nothing is wrong. You have what is euphemistically called the baby blues, although postpartum depression can and does occur and needs to be addressed professionally. The difference between the blues and depression is more a matter of length and depth of feelings and how they affect your life. The postpartum myth that you will glow and bask in the glory of your child is just that, a myth.

You are not perfect. Your partner is not perfect. You are not yourself nor will you be yourself for weeks, if not months. What you need is sleep, more sleep, and then more sleep, and then time. You don't even know that you are in a tunnel, never mind that there is a light at the end of it. Take it moment by moment. You will get through this. You have to. Cry, yell if you must, and then move on.

I cannot for the life of me understand the conspiracy that exists today to make women think that they can and should do this all by themselves. It is impossible to go that long without meaningful sleep and not be irreparably harmed. There existed a time when mothers were home and extended families lived together or quite near to each other. Women tended to mothers because that is what they did. They cared for the baby while the mother slept and handed the baby to their mother to feed as needed. The world is no longer like this. Women work outside the house. Families are often hundreds of miles away, and grandparents often are working and unable to be available for extended periods of time. This is where partners come in. Yes, they are usually still going to work and yes, they do need sleep. But you need sleep as well. Your job tending to this baby is no less important.

Do the best you can to arrange for assistance. Do not judge or reject honest help when it is offered. Eat what is prepared for you. Sleep when time allows. Your baby will survive if someone other than you tends to him or her. Swallow your pride and ask for help when you need it rather than demand it in a tearful or unkind way after you are beyond your wits' end. Your partner and/or your mother or mother-in-law cannot possibly know what you want unless you tell them. They are not mind readers, nor should you expect them to be, "if they loved me."

Above all, remember these two words: "good enough." If the health department has not been called, your house is clean enough. If your baby's crib is not made up exactly as you would have liked, get over it. He or she will sleep just fine. If your mother-in-law holds your baby more than you would like but gives you time to sleep, be happy she is there and cares. If she fixes "sinful" foods that are nutritious, filling, and actually tasty, forget about the calories. Eat and be satisfied. If your husband doesn't swaddle the baby the way you would, who really cares but you? Let him do it. The good and bad news is that there are other people in this universe who can tend to your baby, just not the way you might have liked. You will recover and, believe it or not, you will most likely want to go through this again.

Please note that, as a general rule, women tend to stop when the job is done. Men tend to stop when they are tired. What you would do if you could, how you would do it, and when you would do it are your ideas. Your husband likely will not agree that all of your requests are equally important or even necessary. He will likely have to be asked, often more than once, to do them and will want praise for having done them. This is a reality for many. Your definition of "a job well done" may need to change for a few months. Is it fair? Who knows? But we are talking survival at this point.

Medical Concerns

Breastfeeding

While the opportunity to do this is, for most women, one of the most amazing things one will ever do, the process can take on a life of its own. Feeding your baby every two hours for the first few weeks can be exhausting and time-consuming. Initially, this job is best left to mothers until their supply is well-established. After that, you can pump milk for your baby so that others can share in this task. When you go back to work, you can have a supply in place for your baby if you don't want to use formula.

Breastfeeding rarely goes perfectly the first time. I personally believe there is a conspiracy amongst nurses and lactation consultants to make you think that everything just happens naturally and on cue. They will also tell you that it doesn't hurt if you are doing it right. This is NOT true for first-time moms. Your nipples have never been through anything like a baby suction cupping onto them 12 times a day for 20 minutes at a time. They will hurt at first. That is totally normal.

Also, the reality is that many women do not make enough milk for a number of days, which is why most babies lose some weight in the first few days. If you don't get the anticipated "let down" immediately, don't worry. It often takes more than a day or two for it to happen.

Frequently, the milk does not come in fully at first. It often happens after you leave the hospital. The lactation consultants will look sad and dismal and give you all types of tips to help you in your "failure." Generally, though, after three or four days, there will be 24 hours of hell. Your breasts will get engorged. Your baby will scream and cry to feed and then scream and cry because he or she does not get enough. You may even get a low-grade temperature elevation. This should pass in a day. The milk then comes in, and all is well with the world. (Unless you are over 40, in which case, there is often a decreased ability to make enough milk.)

In the interim, do not be afraid to supplement with formula. Your baby, unless he or she has tongue-tie or some other issue, will not generally abandon the natural urge to nurse. The baby's health is the issue here, not your potentially over-achieving need to succeed at nursing. Whatever works. Second pregnancies, thankfully, are usually much better because you and your body know what you are doing.

Because of the Affordable Care Act, all women are entitled to receive an electric breast pump, which are much more helpful and efficient than hand pumps. The brand that you get and when you receive it (after 28 weeks or after delivery) will depend on your insurance company. For more information on types of pumps, please see the section on breast pumps in the second chapter.

There is a practical issue here, though. If you are nursing every two hours, when do you pump? You can do it between feedings if you wish, but that doesn't leave much time for anything else. What many of my patients have found helpful is to pump one breast while nursing on the other and then switch. The letdown is greater when your baby is nursing, and two tasks are accomplished at the same time.

Some women have difficulty making enough milk for their baby, which can be frustrating to say the least. A visit or two with a lactation specialist can be very helpful here. Also, some babies will simply not take milk from the nipple and insist on bottle-feeding only. Women have taken it upon themselves to pump and feed for extended periods of time under these circumstances. If you wish to do so, that's fine, but the toll it takes on you can be quite high.

Not everyone ends up being able to nourish his or her baby with breast milk. The good news is that there are many excellent quality, if not expensive, formulas available for these situations. No longer are wet nurses needed as in the olden days to keep babies from starving. Your baby can and will thrive and be healthy on formula. Do not let others guilt you into persisting at something that just does not work for you. You are not a failure if breastfeeding doesn't work out. There is no shame in that.

Physical Recovery

You have gone through nine months of a disability of sorts. For that alone, you justifiably deserve a few weeks of rest and recovery. Add to that a long labor and delivery, and, worst of all, a major operative procedure if you had a cesarean section, and you truly do need weeks and weeks to get your body back to some semblance of normal.

On top of all this, you have a baby who needs to be tended to, making it impossible to get 8 to 10 hours of restful sleep in a row each day as you recover. Be kind to yourself. Sleep, or at least rest, when your baby sleeps instead of running around cleaning up and doing laundry. Remember the words "good enough." This is the time to recover, not get your house in order. Being an overachiever myself, I understand that these words are difficult to swallow, but they are true. At least compromise just a little bit on your self-imposed demands. The world truly will not end if you don't fold that load of laundry, and, sadly, it will likely be there for you after you take your nap.

Diet and Exercise

Your diet should include plenty of protein to help replenish what was lost during your labor and delivery and to help you make milk for your baby. What might appear to be excessive amounts of water are necessary to keep you from getting dehydrated and your milk supply from dropping. Continue your prenatal vitamins until your final postpartum visit if you are not nursing. If you are nursing, continue them until about a month after you stop breastfeeding to replenish your stores (perhaps for the next baby?).

Exercise that gives you energy and makes you feel better is all that should be done in the first six to eight weeks. This usually translates into walks after the first two weeks. Start off slowly—stroll, don't power walk. Perhaps you can go around the block a time or two to start. Or have someone take you to a mall where you can walk free from the elements and sit down for something to eat or drink if you tire. There will be plenty of time for working out later, so don't push it.

Getting outside of your house is important for your emotional state at this point. Staying inside in your pajamas or yoga pants, the smell of milk radiating off of you, for days on end will definitely not help with the baby blues. If you can, get away without the baby.

Diastasis Recti

This is a generally benign condition that is defined as a gap between the two sides of the rectus abdominis muscle of more than about two fingerbreadths. In the vast majority of cases, there is no associated morbidity. It is a very common condition. The more babies you have and/or the more weight you gain, the higher the likelihood you will develop it. In reality, only a very small minority of women develop enough weakness in their abdominal muscles from this separation to have difficulty doing things that require core muscle strength, although they might develop back pain as a result.

I mention this because, for some reason, the condition has gotten a lot of buzz on the internet lately. Patients call or come into the office a week or two after having their baby wanting to be checked for diastasis and are referred to a physical therapist or plastic surgeon. This is usually not necessary. When you are finished with your recovery, start concentrating on core body exercises, something that everyone should do anyway. There is really nothing you can do to avoid diastasis.

Mastitis

Mastitis, or the inflammation or infection of the breast, can occur at any time. Symptoms include redness and pain in the affected breast and fever, often to 101- or 102-degrees Fahrenheit. The onset can be quite sudden. You may be feeling well and suddenly start to feel like you've been hit by a truck. Your breast gets sore and your temperature goes up in a matter of hours. If this happens, contact your doctor for treatment with antibiotics to avoid developing an abscess. Nurse or pump from the affected side first. It's okay to do so. Milk is a great culture medium for bacteria, so the breast should be emptied often. Take the antibiotics for the entire recommended time. If you are not feeling somewhat better within 24 hours, call your doctor back and request a follow up.

Skin and Hair Problems

Pregnancy and delivery are very stressful to the body. As a result, a few weeks after delivery, some unwelcome changes may be noted in your skin and hair. Specifically, you may notice blemishes you haven't had before, and you may start to lose hair — a lot of hair. This loss often goes on for weeks or even a few months. The amount can be frightening when you see large clumps in the drain after you wash your hair or a lot of hair on the floor after you comb it. This process is self-limited, meaning it will go away by itself, but it can be unsettling at the time, especially when the body you had before pregnancy has been switched out for another one.

I mention these changes so that you can be reassured that it is common and won't be concerned that there is something seriously wrong with you. You won't like it any bit better, but you can hopefully stop worrying about it.

Weight Loss

Whatever you do, do not stand on the scale immediately after having a baby unless you are a glutton for punishment. Although you may have delivered a 7-pound baby, along with a placenta and amniotic fluid and blood, you generally received a lot of fluid through the IV during your labor. Thus, it is very possible for you to weigh the same—or more—in the days after you have your baby than you did when you entered the hospital. So please, *please*, don't step on that scale.

The postpartum period, especially if you are nursing, is not the time to diet. Your body needs to recover and repair. Making milk for your baby can burn up to 500 calories a day if you are doing it exclusively. There are the lucky vocal few who find it difficult to keep weight on while they are nursing. And then there is everyone else. As with weight gain during pregnancy, calories in and calories burned is a mathematical equation. If you consume more than you use, you will not lose weight.

Generally speaking, by six weeks postpartum, you will have lost all of the weight that you are going to lose naturally. The rest will either have to be painstakingly removed with diet and exercise, or it will sit there until your next pregnancy. In addition, while you nurse, even if you get down to your pre-pregnancy weight, the distribution of that weight will be different; it has an annoying tendency to sit right around your middle. Not fair? No, it is not, but it is very real.

When Will My Period Start Again?

The date of your first menstrual cycle will depend on whether you are nursing (and how much you nurse). If you do not breastfeed, you can expect a cycle about a month after you deliver. If you are exclusively breastfeeding or pumping, you may not get a period until you stop. If you cut back on nursing or are just unlucky, your period can return at any time. This is why breastfeeding should not be counted on as a failsafe method of birth control!

Postpartum Visit

Six weeks after giving birth, most of you will see your doctor for the first time since delivery. (If you had a C-section, you will likely be asked to come in two weeks postpartum for an incision check.) At this visit, you will have your weight checked. You will have a pelvic exam to make sure that your uterus has returned to normal size and that any tears you may have are healed. Your doctor will talk to you about plans for birth control and make an assessment about postpartum depression. (See following section on Hormones and Postpartum Depression.)

Becoming Sexually Active/Birth control

This may be the last thing on your mind when you see your doctor at six weeks because, at this point, when you lie down at night, you will generally and desperately want to go to sleep as soon as possible. However, even the most clueless of men seem to know that six weeks is the time that most women are given the go-ahead to have sex. Remember, nothing happened to their bodies, and they are often anxious to resume normal activities at this point.

If you are nursing, you can use regular birth control pills, but this may result in a decrease in your breast milk. If you are having trouble keeping up with the volume, you could opt to take a progesterone only, or mini-pill. These pills are not quite as effective as the ones that contain estrogen but, when combined with infrequent ovulations while nursing and a general lack of activity due to fatigue, they usually do the trick. When your periods become regular or you stop nursing, switch back to regular pills for better protection.

Many couples opt to use condoms or other forms of physical barriers during this time. Other good options are an IUD or progesterone implant if you are not planning another pregnancy for a few years.

Using breastfeeding alone as birth control is not the best option as women do occasionally ovulate while nursing, even if they do so exclusively. Remember that there are two clinical ways to determine if you have ovulated: either you have a period two weeks later or a baby nine months later.

Hormones and Postpartum Depression[32, 33]

More and more obstetricians are formally testing for depression with a questionnaire (Edinburg Postnatal Depression Scale) at the postpartum visit. This is recommended by the American College of Obstetricians and Gynecologists as well. Certain scores can indicate the likelihood of clinical depression, which, if it exists at this point, should be addressed formally.

Depression is unfortunately an extremely common condition in pregnancy and the postpartum period. When you combine the hormonal changes, sleep deprivation, the physical discomforts, and the realities of the first few weeks, the postpartum period is a perfect set up for this disorder to raise its ugly head. This is especially true if the mother already has an existing predisposition for anxiety and/or depression.

The disability it can cause is immeasurable. Sadness, anger, and fear—and the distance from your baby and loved ones that these emotions cause—can rob you and your family of so much joy during the first several weeks postpartum. At best, it can be an annoyance. At worst, it can be a serious and devastating disorder.

If you, your partner, or your doctor suspect you are suffering from more than just the "baby blues," support groups, counselors, and/or medication are available to help you, depending on your circumstances. Sadly, for many, the stigma, as well as the time and money required to address this very important issue, often keep women from admitting their problems for far too long. There is, and should be, no shame associated with this disorder. If you suffer from it, please avail yourself of any and all assistance. You deserve the help. You have gone through nine months of drama and

---

32. Committee Opinion, 2015.
33. Committee Opinion, 2016.

trauma, as well as a delivery followed by lack of sleep and reality. Let others help you help yourself. You, your baby, and your loved ones deserve this.

Relationships – And Then There Were Three

Parenting Styles

As a couple, you have voluntarily opted to invite another person into your relationship. It can be a glorious addition, but you need to be prepared that there will be changes, some good and some not so good.

There are as many parenting styles as there are individuals. In most cases, with notable exceptions, there are no absolute rights or wrongs when it comes to baby care and child rearing. No matter how you were raised or how much you read or observe with family and friends, there are approaches that work better for some and worse for others. Since this child belongs to the two of you, you will need to work out together how you are going to parent. Be kind and respect each other in this process. It's so easy to do it wrong—and you will do many things wrong, just like every parent—but working together as a team will make things much easier.

Attending parenting classes, preferably before trouble arises, is always a good idea for everyone. Talking about your assumptions and needs in a kind way can go a long way toward healthy parenting as well. Couples and/or individual therapy can also be helpful if needed.

Sexual Relations

The first time you have sex after having a baby may not be a big thrill, especially if you are nursing, because the low estrogen levels can lead to vaginal dryness—and the resultant discomfort. Lubricants can be quite helpful during this time. In addition, you may be surprised that milk may leak, especially with orgasm. For women who are uncomfortable with this, leave your bra on. However, I have gotten the distinct impression from husbands over the years that this matters not one bit to them; they are just happy to be back with their partners.

A glass of wine after nursing your baby might be a helpful option for the first time and make it easier to relax. Make it your partner's job to go out and purchase the most expensive bottle of wine that he cannot afford for this occasion!

There will be some women for whom the above suggestions do not work, especially if they have had an unusually large tear and/or one that takes longer than average to heal completely. They may benefit from the use of an external estrogen cream to help with comfort and lubrication until they finish nursing.

Madonna Complex

This is a term I lovingly use for the postpartum equivalent of the Bridezilla role that many women assume when they are getting married. During pregnancy, especially if it was your first one, everything was about you, how you felt, and what you needed. All of a sudden, this very cute baby takes center stage, and you are no longer the star of the show.

There is bound to be a change in how you view yourself and your role in life and with your partner now that you are a mother. It is difficult when the body you once had is in the repair shop, and the loaner is simply not what you would have chosen. Your stomach is wriggly and loose. Your breasts leak milk. Your hair is falling out. You've got zits. You pee on yourself a little when you cough or sneeze. You are exhausted and often overwhelmed, but this delicious creature you brought home from the hospital brings you such joy. At times, you feel like your baby is all you really need and want. While he or she may be demanding in terms of its needs for feeding and care, your baby loves and needs you in a way that no other human has ever loved or needed you. Your partner's needs and concerns often take second or third place, if they even rank at all, to this amazing being. Some of that is necessary and fair given the demands, but do mind that you don't take things to the extreme.

You will not always look at your breasts as for the baby only and not for touch by your partner. When you stop nursing, you will get your libido back. Until then, you may feel as if you have been temporarily castrated, which, biologically, you have, since your ovaries have been suppressed. For a moment, though, if you can, think of how you would feel if your partner suddenly lost all interest in you sexually. You say that you would be okay with that, but would you really? Would your feelings not be hurt even just a little bit? Yes, he is a grown man and should understand, but he is also only human.

You will not always think of your partner as someone who doesn't get it in terms of the bazillion extra things you feel now need to be done and when. You are going to want him there for you in the future (especially if you want another child). If you dismiss him too severely or for too long, some of the fire will permanently be put out of the relationship. Know that babies never make a bad relationship better, and they often test, to the very limits, a good and solid one.

This is not to say that partners don't have the responsibility of understanding the pressures you are under. Many men are hurt by the fact that they don't get as much attention as they did before the baby. Well, there are three of you now, and your wife is only one person. Her life has changed. Yours must change as well. Yes, you have commuted and worked eight-plus hours and missed your baby, but your wife has not just been sitting at home eating bonbons and watching your baby sleep. You cannot expect to come home to a spotless house, a delicious dinner, and a wife who magically turns into a sex kitten when the baby goes to sleep. That just isn't going to happen. In fact, my experience has been that the majority of time that men stay home with the baby, they view their task as simply to keep the lions from eating their little one. Their wife comes home to a trashed house and an irritable partner and is handed a screaming baby with a soiled diaper before she can change out of her work clothes. So, partners, when you come home in the evenings, consider that perhaps the sexiest things you can do are clean the dinner dishes or take the baby and tell your wife to go take a bubble bath.

Years ago, I knew a nurse who married someone much younger than her. Before marriage, he told her that he enjoyed sex and wanted to have it on a daily basis, if not more. Her response was, "Make me want it." I admire her for that, as did he. She regularly received poems or loving texts from him. He would show up at the end of her shift with flowers and keys to a hotel room. He understood that it was his job to seduce her, not her duty to have sex with him because he was her husband.

You were a team of two before. Now you are a team of three. Embrace this and grow with it and each other.

Endnote/Author's Note

Much has changed since the 1980s when I started my career and had my children. At that time, the first brave group of women who were working outside of the house began to have babies and return to work. The world was not ready for this phenomenon. Maternity leaves were six weeks of your previously earned sick and vacation time or leave without pay. Your job was not necessarily guaranteed if you stayed away longer than six weeks, so many did not. Daycare centers were few and far between. There was no such thing as after-school care at your child's elementary school. If you wanted your child to be watched after school, you had to get a sitter or someone to take them to one of the local centers if you could not leave your job to do so. Summer camps were for those who could be available to drop their children off and pick them up before and after rush hours. In other words, they were for stay-at-home moms.

Now many women regularly get up to 10 or 12, and in some cases, 16 weeks of paid maternity leave. Sometimes spouses get leave as well, not for having the baby, of course, but for childcare. And they can now use that leave without the risk of being seen as "not partner material."

Pumping stations are available in many workplaces, airports, and other public areas other than in bathrooms. Public restrooms have parent rooms with changing tables.

Goldman Sachs will express deliver frozen breast milk to the homes of their employees who have to be away from their babies for meetings and conferences out-of-town. Google and other companies pay for egg freezing, aka fertility preservation, for their valued employees in their 30s.

While much more needs to be done in terms of accepting that nature has given women a limited window in which to reproduce and that women rightfully choose to do so at a time when their careers are taking off, I credit millennials for the impetus for these changes. Good for you!

I also credit millennials with having a much greater understanding of the childbirth and parenting processes. In general, the more knowledge, the better—to a point, anyway. I once had a patient who was a nuclear physicist. At her last visit before delivery, I asked if she had any questions. Her response? "I know everything there is to know about having a baby." Suffice it to say that her introduction to reality was challenging, to say the least.

There can be a dark side to all of this knowledge though. The dead baby websites are the perfect example. While seeking perfection, millennials often fear the worst and look for it. I can't begin to tell you how many of my patients have called, panic-stricken, after looking at these awful sites. Even on Web MD, a tiny, inconsequential symptom can be made to look as if you or your baby will die soon if it is not tended to immediately. In general, it's best to stay away from these sites, but, I'm told, it's like a train wreck: you just can't stop yourself from looking at it.

An oft-asked question by my patients at the end of their prenatal visit was, "What do I need to worry about next?" This as opposed to, "What sorts of things can I expect in the next month?" This need to "horriblize" is sadly rampant in today's culture. I can only recommend that you control what you can control and accept that which you cannot without obsessing about it. Above all else, stop going online so much!

I have a cup on my desk that says, "Please do not confuse your Google research for my medical degree." Many today tend to do just that. While I could have gone to law school or become a CPA, I would never presume to go to my attorney or accountant and bullishly insist that I know more than they do about their field. Nor would I imply that my attorney is somehow working to put me in jail, or my accountant is trying to send me into bankruptcy. This attitude, however, is not that uncommon for some who feel they know more than their doctors simply because of their "research," which is often not evidence-based.

Worse yet, these women are often convinced that their doctor is likely to cause harm to them or their child with vaccines, medications, and medical procedures. While it is true that, in the past, medical professionals often let patients down by being, at times, arrogant, self-serving individuals who placed themselves in the middle of the narrative rather than the patient, that is generally no longer the case. "Trust me, I'm a doctor" is not good enough these days for a reason. Evidence-based practice is what is required.

Do your research, please. Ask all of the questions you need to ask and choose a doctor who you feel comfortable with, whose philosophies match yours. Believe it or not, your doctor is there to help you through this process.

Will your child be absolutely gorgeous, brilliant, and the most successful person on the planet? Probably not. Will you love him or her more than you ever thought it possible to love another human being in the world? YES. That is the beauty of this whole thing. You have created a perfectly imperfect human who you get to hold and love and guide through the coming years and share the good, the bad, and the ugly with. I don't know many parents who have regretted making that choice.

Hopefully, after reading my book you will have come to understand that we are all on the same team with one common goal: to provide you with a safe pregnancy and the delivery of a healthy baby to a healthy mom. It's an honor to have done so for so many years.

I thank you for taking the time to read my musings and hope you have picked up a couple of Dr. J's pearls along the way. I wish you the best of luck in your journey!

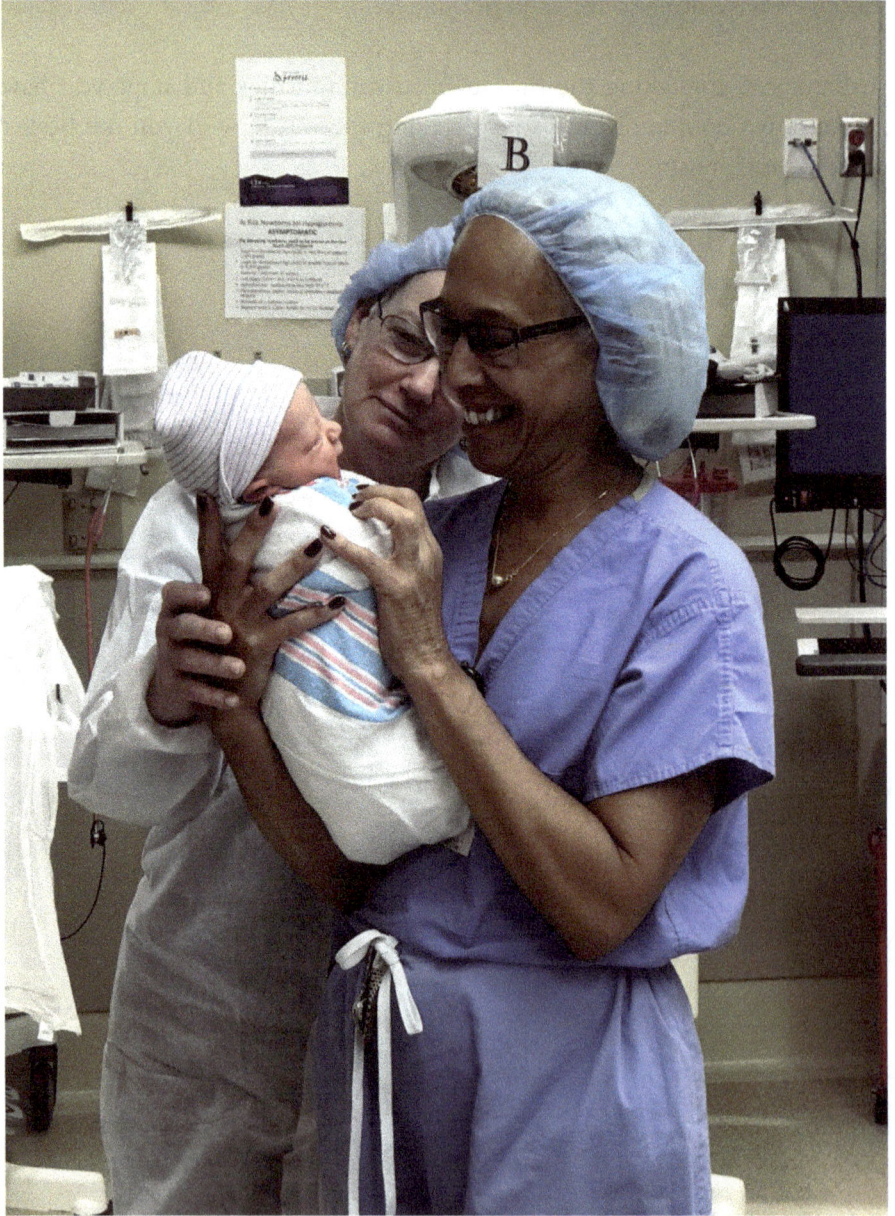

Me holding Jack David, the last baby of my career

Acknowledgments

To my patients, who have taught me more than I could ever have learned from a textbook or journal article.

To Katie (Merkel) O'Hare, Michael O'Hare, and Diane Merkel for granting me the privilege of delivering Jack David, my last baby and their first child and grandchild, and the incentive to put my thoughts and experiences to pen.

To Atlantic Publishing Group, who took a chance on my very first book.

To Danielle Lieneman, a spectacular editor, who "got" what I wanted to say and how I wanted to say it.

To Marcel Trindade, my illustrator and now friend, who also "got" what I wanted to say and how I wanted to portray it.

To Jeff Anthony, my life partner, whose gentle, but firmly persistent, encouragement guided me to write this book.

To Zoe Alpert, my medical assistant, whose kind, but insistent, red pen helped prepare my draft for presentation.

To Sarah (Johnson) Conway, my daughter and forever partner-in-crime and best friend; Susannah Kearns, my medical guru; Cheryl Somarriba, my sister and amazing OB nurse, and her daughter, Stephanie Huffman, my unofficial proofreaders—for their editorial assistance.

This book would not have been possible without any of you.

Glossary

Aerobic activity: Exercise that requires the use of oxygen; also called cardio

AFP, AFP Plus: Alpha FetoProtein blood tests done at 16 weeks to look for evidence of defects in the spinal cord and brain

Amniocentesis: A test performed in the 16th week of pregnancy that involves inserting a needle under ultrasonic guidance into the amniotic sac to obtain fluid containing fetal cells

Amniotic fluid: The fluid that surrounds a baby in the uterus

Anatomy Scan: Sonogram done at 20 weeks to look for structural abnormalities in the baby

Apgar Score: A test given to babies at one and five minutes of life to determine if extra or emergency care is required

Basal body temperature charts: Where you record your morning temperature every day immediately upon waking and before having anything to eat or drink; can be used to gain information about your ovulation

Body Mass Index (BMI): A calculated measure of body fat that is based on height and weight. Normal is up to 25; 25 to 30 is considered overweight; 30 to 40 is considered obese; and over 40 is considered morbidly obese

Cell-Free Fetal DNA: DNA from the fetus that circulates in the maternal blood stream and can be used to determine if the baby has a chromosomal or genetic abnormality; can also determine if the fetus is a boy or a girl

Cerclage: A stitch placed in the cervix to keep it closed during pregnancy

Cesarean Delivery: A surgical procedure to deliver a baby through an abdominal incision rather than through the vagina

Chorionic villi sampling: A test that samples cells destined to develop into placental tissue

Conceive: To become pregnant

Cone Biopsy: Procedure using a scalpel to remove a cone-shaped segment of the cervix that contains precancerous cells

Congenital abnormalities: Birth defects

Cord Blood Banking: Collection of fetal stem cells from the umbilical cord after delivery to be stored for potential future use

Core body temperature: The temperature at which the body operates

Corpus luteum: Collection of cells in the ovary that produce progesterone to support a developing pregnancy

Diastasis recti: A gap between the two sides of the rectus abdominis muscles (paired muscles that run the length of the anterior abdominal wall) of more than about two centimeters (2.54 cm to an inch)

Dilation and Curettage (D&C): Procedure to remove tissue from the uterus; the cervix is dilated, and the tissue remove by suction or scraping

Doula: A lay birthing coach

Ectopic pregnancy: A pregnancy outside of the uterine cavity, which cannot survive, and can result in catastrophic bleeding

Embryologic dating: Pregnancy dating based on the date of conception or ovulation

Endometriosis: A disease where glands that normally line the uterine cavity grow in other places in the pelvis

Fertility specialist: Physician who specializes in individuals who have difficulty getting pregnant

Folic acid: B complex vitamin

Forceps: A metal instrument shaped like a large spoon that can be applied to a baby's head to facilitate delivery

Gestational Diabetes: Pregnancy-associated glucose intolerance, or diabetes

Glucose Tolerance Test (GTT): Test done to determine if someone with an abnormal screen for diabetes has diabetes

Health Maintenance Organization (HMO): Health insurance plan that provides all of your care within a network of providers who accept your insurance

Human chorionic gonadotropic (HCG): Pregnancy hormone level

Immunocompromised state: Weakened immune system

In vitro fertilization: A procedure where egg and sperm are united outside of the body and then transferred into the uterus

Incompetent cervix: A weakened cervix that dilates painlessly in the second trimester of pregnancy, leading to delivery before the fetus is viable

Laborist: Obstetrician who works full-time at a hospital

Loop Electrical Excision Procedure (LEEP): A procedure using electrical cautery to remove precancerous cells from the cervix

Luteinizing hormone (LH): A hormone produced by the pituitary gland to stimulate the release of an egg (ovulation)

Mastitis: Inflammation or infection of the breast

Meconium: Fetal stool

Methylmercury: A poisonous form of mercury

Multips: Those who have had at least one delivery

Neural tube defects: Abnormalities of the spinal cord and brain such as spina bifida or meningomyelocele

Nondisjunction: The failure of chromosomes to separate normally when the nucleus of the cell divides, resulting in an abnormal distribution of chromosomes in the newly formed cells

Obstetrical dating: Pregnancy dating based on the first day of the last menstrual period

Ovulate: Release an egg from your ovary

Parvovirus B19: A relatively harmless virus in children that can cause serious problems for your baby, especially if you are exposed to it in the first trimester; known more commonly as slapped cheek syndrome

Patent ductus arteriosus: A defect that involves the opening of two blood vessels that lead to the heart and can lead to heart failure and elevated pressure in the lungs of infants

Perineal Massage: Stretching of the muscles surrounding the vaginal opening to prepare for childbirth

Pertussis: Virus that causes whooping cough

Pessary: Plastic device placed in the vagina to hold the cervix in place

Pitocin: Commercial version of oxytocin, which is produced by the brain, to strengthen or initiate contractions of the uterus to induce or augment labor, or after delivery to reduce bleeding

Placenta: The organ that supplies oxygen and nutrients to a growing baby

Polycystic ovarian syndrome (PCOS): A disease associated with multiple ovarian cysts and irregular menstrual cycles

Postpartum depression: Clinical depression that occurs in the postpartum period

Preferred Provider Organization (PPO): Insurance plan that has a number of participating providers who accept your insurance

Prenatal vitamins: Vitamins specifically designed to address a pregnant woman's needs

Primips: Those who are pregnant for the first time

Progesterone: A hormone produced by the ovaries to support a developing pregnancy

Tongue tie: A condition that limits the range of motion of an infant's tongue

Toxoplasmosis: A disease caused by the Toxoplasma gondii parasite; frequently found in cat feces

Unrecognized pregnancies: Positive pregnancy tests without the development of a recognizable fetus.

Vacuum: A suction device placed on the fetal scalp to facilitate delivery.

Pregnancy Timeline

LMP: First day of your last menstrual period

Day 14: Probable time of ovulation; day 5 after embryo implantation if conceived via IVF

Day 28: When period would be expected; first likely time for a positive home pregnancy test

6 weeks (from the first day of your LMP): First possible time to see the fetal heart beating on ultrasound

6–10 weeks: First visits to OB to confirm viable pregnancy, get genetic counseling and prenatal labs

Prenatal labs include:

- Blood type and antibody screen
- Rubella titer (are you immune to German measles?)
- Varicella titer (are you immune to chicken pox?)
- Blood count (are you anemic?)

- Urinalysis and urine culture (urinary tract infections are common in pregnancy and have been associated with pre-term labor and/or the development of kidney infections)

- Pap smear (if indicated)

- Sexually transmitted diseases screening (syphilis, gonorrhea, and chlamydia are required by law in most states)

- Hepatitis B (recommended by the American Academy of Pediatricians)

- HIV/AIDS (recommended by the American College of Obstetricians and Gynecologists and the CDC)

There are other optional labs and tests that you may need to take if you fit the appropriate high-risk profile. Please discuss with your provider.

Optional labs and tests:

- Parvovirus, Firth or Slap Disease

- Toxoplasmosis (for cat owners)

- Cystic fibrosis screen

- Jewish panel screen (Tay-Sachs disease, Canavan's, and familial dysautonomia screen)

- Sickle trait screen

- Thalassemia screen

- General or universal panel for various recessive genetic disorders, and a finger stick for Ultra-Screen test

10 weeks:

- Cell-free fetal DNA testing for chromosomal abnormalities and fetal gender

- Finger stick for Ultrascreen test

- Fetal heartbeat heard with a doptone

12 weeks: Ultrasound for Ultra-Screen, to be combined with finger stick from 10-week visit

13 weeks: Beginning of the second trimester; all major organ systems have been formed and the risk for miscarriage is now very low

16 weeks: Sonogram and blood work for AFP, AFP Plus, or tetra screen to look for any increased risk for chromosomal abnormalities or potential problems in the third trimester; uterus palpable halfway from the top of the pubic bone to the belly button

20 weeks: Uterus palpable at the belly bottom; anatomy screen ultrasound

24 weeks: One-hour glucola (diabetes) screen; additional labs include blood count (anemia screen), antibody screen, and RhoGAM shot if mom is Rh negative to protect the baby, and syphilis screen; fetal movement begins to be apparent; baby could survive outside the womb; second trimester ends

36 weeks: Repeat STD screen, +/- HIV titer, blood count (last anemia screen), Beta strep, vaginal and rectal culture (approximately 10 to 30 percent of women are carriers of this bacteria which has been associated with serious infections in the newborn. Mothers who test positive at any time will be treated in labor with intravenous antibiotics.)

38–42 weeks: full term; the vast majority of women will deliver in this time frame

Works Cited

The American College of Obstetricians and Gynecologists. *2018 Compendium of Selected Publications.* The American College of Obstetricians and Gynecologists, 2018, pp. 2–9.

Baskett, Thomas F., and Fritz Nagele. "Naegele's Rule: a Reappraisal." *BJOG: An International Journal of Obstetrics and Gynaecology*, vol. 107, no. 11, 2000, pp. 1433–1435., doi:10.1111/j.1471-0528.2000.tb11661.x.

Centers for Disease Control and Prevention. "National Survey of Family Growth." National Center for Health Statistics. 26 June 2019. www.cdc.gov. Accessed 9 February 2019.

Cleveland Clinic. "Female Reproductive System." Cleveland Clinic. 19 January 2019. www.myclevelandclinic.org. Accessed 1 February 2019.

"Committee Opinion No. 82: Management of Herpes in Pregnancy." *Obstetrics & Gynecology*, vol. 109, no. 6, 2007, pp. 1489–1498.

"Committee Opinion No. 130: Prediction and Prevention of Preterm Birth." *Obstetrics & Gynecology*, vol. 120, no. 4, October 2012, pp. 964–973., doi: 10.1097/AOG.0b013e3182723b1b.

"Committee Opinion No. 462: Moderate Caffeine Consumption During Pregnancy." *Obstetrics & Gynecology*, vol. 116, no. 2, Part 1, 2010, pp. 467–468., doi:10.1097/aog.0b013e3181eeb2a1.

"Committee Opinion No. 495: Vitamin D: Screening and Supplementation During Pregnancy." *Obstetrics & Gynecology*, vol. 118, no. 1, 2011, pp. 197–198., doi:10.1097/aog.0b013e318227f06b.

"Committee Opinion No. 548: Weight Gain During Pregnancy." *Obstetrics & Gynecology*, vol. 121, 2013, pp. 210–212.

"Committee Opinion No. 630: Screening for Perinatal Depression." *Obstetrics & Gynecology*, vol. 125, no. 5, May 2015, pp. 1268–1271.

"Committee Opinion No. 648: Umbilical Cord Blood Banking." *Obstetrics & Gynecology*, vol. 126, no. 6, December 2015, pp. 127–129., doi: 10.1097/AOG.0000000000001212.

"Committee Opinion No. 666: Optimizing Postpartum Care." *Obstetrics & Gynecology*, vol. 127, no. 6, June 2016, pp. 187–192., doi: 10.1097/AOG.0000000000001487.

"Committee Opinion No. 684: Delayed Umbilical Cord Clamping After Birth." *Obstetrics & Gynecology*, vol. 129, no. 1, January 2017, pp.5–10., doi: 10.1097/AOG.0000000000001860.

Federal Register. "Content and Format of Labeling for Human Prescription Drug and Biological Products; Requirements for Pregnancy and Lactation Labeling." *Federal Register: Proposed Rules*, vol. 73, no. 104, 29 May 2008. www.gpo.gov. Accessed 9 February 2019.

Fox, Nathan S. "Dos and Dont's in Pregnancy: Truths and Myths." *Obstetrics & Gynecology*, vol. 131, no. 4, April 2018, pp. 713–721.

Gilbert, Ruth and Eskild Petersen. "Toxoplasmosis and pregnancy." 26 November 2018. www.uptodate.com. Accessed 9 February 2019.

Greer, Frank R., et al. "The Effects of Early Nutritional Interventions on the Development of Atopic Disease in Infants and Children: The Role of Maternal Dietary Restriction, Breastfeeding, Hydrolyzed Formulas, and Timing of Introduction of Allergenic Complementary Foods." *Pediatrics*, vol. 143, no. 4, 2019, pp. 1–11, doi: 10.1542/peds.2019-0281.

Hook, Ernest B., et al. "Chromosomal Abnormality Rates at Amniocentesis and in Live-Born Infants." *Jama*, vol. 249, no. 15, 1983, p. 2034., doi:10.1001/jama.1983.03330390038028.

Houston, Rickie. "Average Cost of Having a Baby in 2018." SmartAsset. 21 August 2019. www.smartasset.com. Accessed 9 April 2019.

The Jewish Agency for Israel. "Be Fruitful and Multiply." The Jewish Agency for Israel. 28 August 2005. archive.jewishagency.org. Accessed 9 February 2019.

JEWNIVERSE. "What The Talmud Talks About When It Talks About Sex." Jewish Telegraphic Agency. 30 March 2016. www.jta.org. Accessed 9 February 2019.

life'sDHA. "DHA Facts." life'sDHA. 2018. www.lifesdha.com. Accessed 9 February 2019.

Mittendorf, R., et al. "The Length of Uncomplicated Human Gestation." *Obstetrics & Gynecology*, vol. 75, no. 6, June 1990, pp. 929–932.

Office of NIH History. "A Timeline of Pregnancy Testing." National Institutes of Health. December 2003. history.nih.gov. Accessed 9 February 2019.

"Practice Bulletin No. 151: Cytomegalovirus, Parvovirus B19, Varicella Zoster, and Toxoplasmosis in Pregnancy." *Obstetrics & Gynecology*, vol. 127, no. 2, 2016, doi:10.1097/aog.0000000000001280.

Toby, Mekeisha Madden. "Can a Fever During Pregnancy Harm My Baby?" healthline. 11 January 2018. www.healthline.com. Accessed 9 April 2019.

U.S. Food and Drug Administration. "Advice about Eating Fish." U.S. Food and Drug Administration. 2 July 2019. www.fda.gov. Accessed 1 February 2019.

U.S. Food and Drug Administration. "Food Safety for Moms-to-Be: Educator's Resource Guide." U.S. Food and Drug Administration. 2017. www.fda.gov. Accessed 1 February 2019.

U.S. Food and Drug Administration. "Pregnancy and Lactation Labeling (Drugs) Final Rule." U.S. Food and Drug Administration. 28 June 2018. www.fda.gov. Accessed 9 February 2019.

About the Author

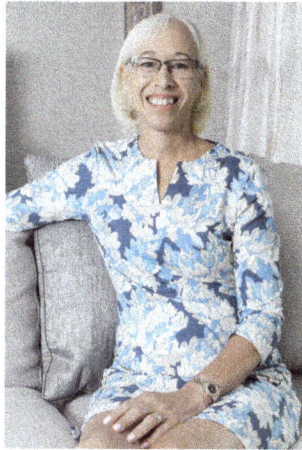

Dr. Heather Johnson is a senior partner at Reiter, Hill, Johnson and Nevin, with offices in Washington, D.C., Chevy Chase, Maryland, and Falls Church, Virginia, where she has been since 2001. Dr. Johnson is an actively practicing gynecologist and retired obstetrician after delivering babies for 40 years.

She attended Yale University School of Medicine and trained at the Walter Reed Army Medical Center in Washington, D.C. She has two children, Clarion Johnson III, JD and Sarah Conway, MD along with one grand-daughter, Harper, and another on the way.

She can be reached at writedrj@gmail.com.

www.ingramcontent.com/pod-product-compliance
Lightning Source LLC
Chambersburg PA
CBHW072206270326
41930CB00011B/2545